CRACKING THE BODY TRANSFORMATION CODE

5 PROVEN WAYS TO A NEW YOU!

CRACKING THE BODY TRANSFORMATION CODE

5 PROVEN WAYS TO A NEW YOU!

SIZWE GUMEDE

First published in 2021, Johannesburg, South Africa

ISBN 978-0-620-89507-1

Co-author Gloria Britain
Photographs Dayle Solomon
Copy Editor Alma Green
Layout and Design Flamescreation

ABOUT THE AUTHOR

Sizwe Gumede has made his name as a Personal Trainer, Yoga Teacher and Virtual Health Coach. With over fifteen years' experience in the health and fitness industry, he is known by his clients as a Personal Trainer who commits to personalising his services to achieve results through consistent inspiration and motivation, taking great interest in each of his clients.

He has mentored new Personal Trainers joining the industry, anchoring them as they take their first steps into the world of personal training.

Sizwe has spent years formulating and testing his unique approach to health and fitness which is contained in the five codes for body transformation.

This is his first book.

DEDICATION

An idea is only an idea until it has been tested.

I dedicate this book to my many clients who experimented with and tested the Five Codes for Body Transformation. With your feedback and collaboration, this knowledge can now be made available to more people who want to lead healthy and active lives.

You are the real heroes of this book, and the future of health and fitness.

ACKNOWLEDGEMENTS

Writing a book is more challenging than I thought it would be, and more rewarding than I could have ever imagined.

Firstly, I'd like to thank all my clients who have given me the opportunity to take them through their Body Transformation journey. You have been the inspiration and the impetus for me writing *Cracking the Body Transformation Code -Five Proven Ways to A New You!*

My appreciation goes to all of you who have gone through my programme and have trusted me and my method of Body Transformation. I have learned as much from you as I hope you have learned from me. Writing this book would not have been possible without your feedback and your willingness to commit to all the various aspects of the programme.

A special thanks to my friends, Amy Da Silva, Dawie Van Vuuren, Tiffany Smith, Natasha Goring, Lia and Dox Lentzakis, Tebogo Serobatse Ngxande and William Ngwenya. Your friendship and encouragement have led me to stepping into new spaces.

A sincere thanks to colleagues and fellow Personal Trainers who helped me gain new and exciting insights into health and fitness. I particularly thank, Liezel Best, Evans Malivhusa, Letitia Kleynhans, Carel Grobler, Kopano Mokhele, Enhle Thwala - Personal Trainers, and bio kineticists, Erin Karam and Shaun Mackay.

My appreciation to Dayle Solomon for taking the photographs. You were the right person at the right time.

Having an idea and turning it into a book is as hard as it sounds. The experience has been both challenging and rewarding. To Gloria Britain, my client, who collaborated and supported the conceptualising process, and co-authored the book. We did it!

My deepest gratitude to you all! Without you, this book would still have been just an idea.

IN PRAISE OF THE FIVE CODES FOR BODY TRANSFORMATION PROGRAMME

Let me start by saying I feel very fortunate to have Sizwe as my personal trainer. I could not have chosen a better trainer. Sizwe is very good at what he does and with his advice on what to eat and how to train. Training with Sizwe is very rewarding. I feel like a million dollars after a training session with Sizwe. He takes his job very seriously. Every session is different. I've learnt a lot. He has a great personality, built extremely well, and he takes great interest in his clients, and he has become a friend to me. **Sharon**

❖

I was a point where I had to face that working on my own was not going to get me results. Everything I did was getting me nowhere slowly. With Sizwe, I lost a total of 17kg going through the Body Transformation Programme. I improved my Midmar Mile swim time by 4 minutes and 13 seconds in the first year I trained with him, which I thought was impossible. I have learned how important Support and Accountability is and how it can change your mindset and keep you focussed. Sizwe's holistic programme helped me make lifestyle changes. It's the best thing I could have done. Thanks, Sizwe… as I always say – you're da best! **Gloria**

❖

I have been training with Sizwe for just over a year and have noticed a huge difference in my physique, energy and stress levels. He is a motivational trainer who is dedicated to his clients. The training sessions are varied, challenging, and push you to the limit. I recommend Sizwe as a personal trainer due to his experience, great personality, and ability to work wonders! **Leigh**

❖

I have been training with Sizwe Gumede during my pregnancy and for a couple of months now since giving birth. His exercise routines are easy to follow and never boring, which keeps me motivated. The yoga classes are relaxing and enjoyable. My body is starting to show the benefits of regular exercise, and I feel healthier than ever. Sizwe is a fantastic trainer who inspires one to push oneself a little bit further every time. **Karin**

❖

Sizwe is good at motivating the class and has a good energy about him. He always gives us tips on how to eat healthily. When departing from his classes, you definitely feel like you have had a good work out. When looking back at myself before starting classes with him and comparing it with myself today, I have seen a positive change in my body, which makes me feel good about myself. **Andrea**

❖

Sizwe knows his stuff. I have an old hip injury, and I have been seen a bio kineticist for many years. She has helped a great deal with healing the injury. I decided to consult Sizwe to give me additional exercises to add to the healing process. He consulted the bio kineticist and worked out a programme for me. His exercises have given me greater strength and flexibility. **Laurentia**

FOREWORD
BY GLORIA BRITAIN

I met Sizwe in March 2019. This was to be the start of a challenging yet rewarding health and fitness encounter . Being in your fifties is not for sissies! My weight was increasing year on year and no matter how I fasted, drank more water, juiced, detoxed, and exercised, I would lose between 2-3 kgs and then, put it back again.

My turning point came when I signed up with Sizwe. This was my first experience with a Personal Trainer, and the thought of having someone to coach me through a health and fitness process was reassuring.

One of the first things I learned was to eat to fuel my body so that my metabolism could function better. This was one of my toughest mind shifts to make as I believed that I had to eat as little as possible to lose weight.

Sizwe gradually built up my fitness levels. He patiently counted the repetition, giving me breaks when I needed them, and making sure I was working hard enough.

Stress comes with the territory of living and working in a city like Johannesburg. Working out with Sizwe helped me to develop a positive attitude. By the end of the sessions, I was reenergised. My evenings transformed into quality time. I now relax, read, reflect on the day and problem solve.

I like to think of myself as mentally tough and able to self-motivate. Well, I learnt how much better it is to have support through this programme. Sizwe, who also virtually coached and sent reminders by Whatsapp, short video clips on social media, kept me on track. The best part was his empathy for when I wasn't feeling my best self – he knew just how to keep me going and pushed me just enough to keep me motivated.

Working with Sizwe is amazing !

I am more mentally alert and focussed, feel strong and confident in my body, have less stiffness and aching muscles. My sleep is good, quality sleep and wake up refreshed. I've started making better food choices and a cheat day doesn't appeal to me. I can see how my body is transforming and see more muscular definition – which I am excited about. I have adopted a new lifestyle. When I don't work out, I feel as if there is something missing in my day. (but I'm not a fanatic yet)

I can look back to my old self now and see where I started from and the progress is awesome.

I've learnt so much more about the five codes after working with Sizwe on this book as his co-author. Our work together has been an awesome partnership of learning and growing.

Gloria Britain
Co-author and Client

CONTENTS

INTRODUCTION

Hi, I am Sizwe Gumede, a full-time Personal Trainer, Yoga Teacher, and a Virtual Health Coach.

My life's purpose is to help people to transform their bodies - whether it is to lose or gain weight, build muscle, or get fit. I believe that everyone can have a great quality of life by developing and maintaining a healthy lifestyle.

There are two reasons I have written this book. Firstly, I want to share my personal experience with Body Transformation so that you won't have to experience the same challenges I did when I started. Secondly, I want to share my professional knowledge with you to educate you about health and fitness. By introducing you to my unique and holistic programme – The Five Codes to Body Transformation, I hope that you will be encouraged to start on a journey that will give you a new outlook on life.

Over the past fifteen years, I have worked with people to get them healthy, fit, manage stress, and transform their bodies through using this programme.

I have followed this programme myself as my daily health and fitness practice, so I have tried it, and I know it is effective.

In this book, you'll learn what the Body Transformation codes are and how to use them.

By now, I'm sure you are wondering - "what is a code, and how does it work?" So lets begin.

Think about all your technological devices – your phone, watch, car - almost every device is a computer and relies on coding. Each number or letter programmed or coded tells the computer to do something in its memory.

By themselves, computers don't know how to do anything. It is the programmer's job to give the computer instructions through coding it. You type in what you want it to do; the coder turns it into language the computer understands, then the computer does it.

In the same way, our bodies also have to be coded for it to perform at its best.

What are the Five Body Transformation Codes?
The five codes of my programme are a holistic way of getting fit and healthy.

The five codes are made up of 20% Food and Hydration, 20% Movement, 20% Stress Management, 20% Rest and Recovery, and 20% Support and Accountability, which makes up 100% of the programme.

Each of the codes complements the other and works in an integrated way. Each of them is equally important to transform your body successfully.

I have taken many people through this programme over my years of being a Personal Trainer. The results and successes of this method has been proven.

These clients are just like anyone else. They have had to overcome the challenges of not succeeding with other attempts. They have had to overcome the fear of failing again but still take the action of following this programme. This is essential for you to know because if they could do it, you can too!

Each of the chapters will teach you about these five codes so that you get to understand them and learn how to code your body to lead you to a new you.

The first step in having a successful body transformation is:

DECIDING WHAT YOU WANT!

If you don't have a clear image in your mind of your endpoint, you will not reach your goals. And even if you do reach them, you may feel the satisfaction because you won't know that you have reached it.

The best way to change anything, is to have a plan. The first chapter of this book is about getting started. You have to know where you are in order for you to plan for where you would like to be. I will take you through a step-by-step process that will help you clarify your health and fitness goals.

Only when you have set your goals will you be ready to start your body transformation programme.

In the second chapter, I will explain the first code – nutrition and hydration, which counts for 20% of the programme.

There are many theories and ideas about nutrition and hydration for health and fitness. I'm going to explain just five of these: Eating high-quality food, How frequently you should eat, Macronutrients, Calorie intake, and Hydration.

To transform your body- you have to get moving. I take you through the second code in chapter three, which is 20% of the body transformation codes - movement. I'm going to tell you about movement generally, and then give you some specific body transformation exercises, stretches, and also, some isometric exercises. There are many ways to move. Functional movements are movements we do as a normal part of our day, like walking and doing activities around the house like gardening and cleaning. I will touch on all of these.

Next, in chapter four, you are going to learn about the third code, stress management, which is the next 20 % of the programme. I will start by looking at what stress management is and some techniques for managing stress through relaxation prayer, meditation, and hobbies.

I use a particular yoga practice, Yoga Nidra, as a stress management technique which I will share with you.

Chapter five is all about rest and recovery, both are important aspects of your body transformation programme. Although they may seem like the same thing, they are different. The first aspect is managing your body's recovery after exercising, and the second is sleep – shutting down the body, mind, and spirit so that you can refresh and reset.

The most important reason for including rest and recovery in your programme is to give yourself the appropriate time to rest, refresh and re-energise. This is just as important as all the other codes and something not often taken seriously enough in a health and fitness programme. This is another 20% of the programme.

Chapter six is about Support and Accountability and is the last 20 % of the programme. It is one of the most powerful codes for reaching your goals. With both support to stay on track and accountability to measure and evaluate where you are, you stand a much better chance of succeeding than trying to do it all by yourself.

Bringing all five codes together will need patience, time, commitment, and grit! It has taken me more than ten years to understand each of these codes of this programme, and how they complement each other - and still, I work on them every day.

When you start out, you may find that some of the codes will be easier for you to practice than others. Commit to the ones that challenge you, don't avoid them. Don't be despondent if you are working hard on three of them, but the other two just seem to be too hard to include. Don't give up; it will be worth your while in the end!

"Accept the challenge so that you may feel the exhilaration of victory."
George Patton

YOU can transform your body. With this book, you have taken the first step - well done!

My goal is to help 1 000 000 people reach their health and fitness potential in my lifetime- I hope you will be one of them.

Sizwe Gumede
Dedicated to your Fitness

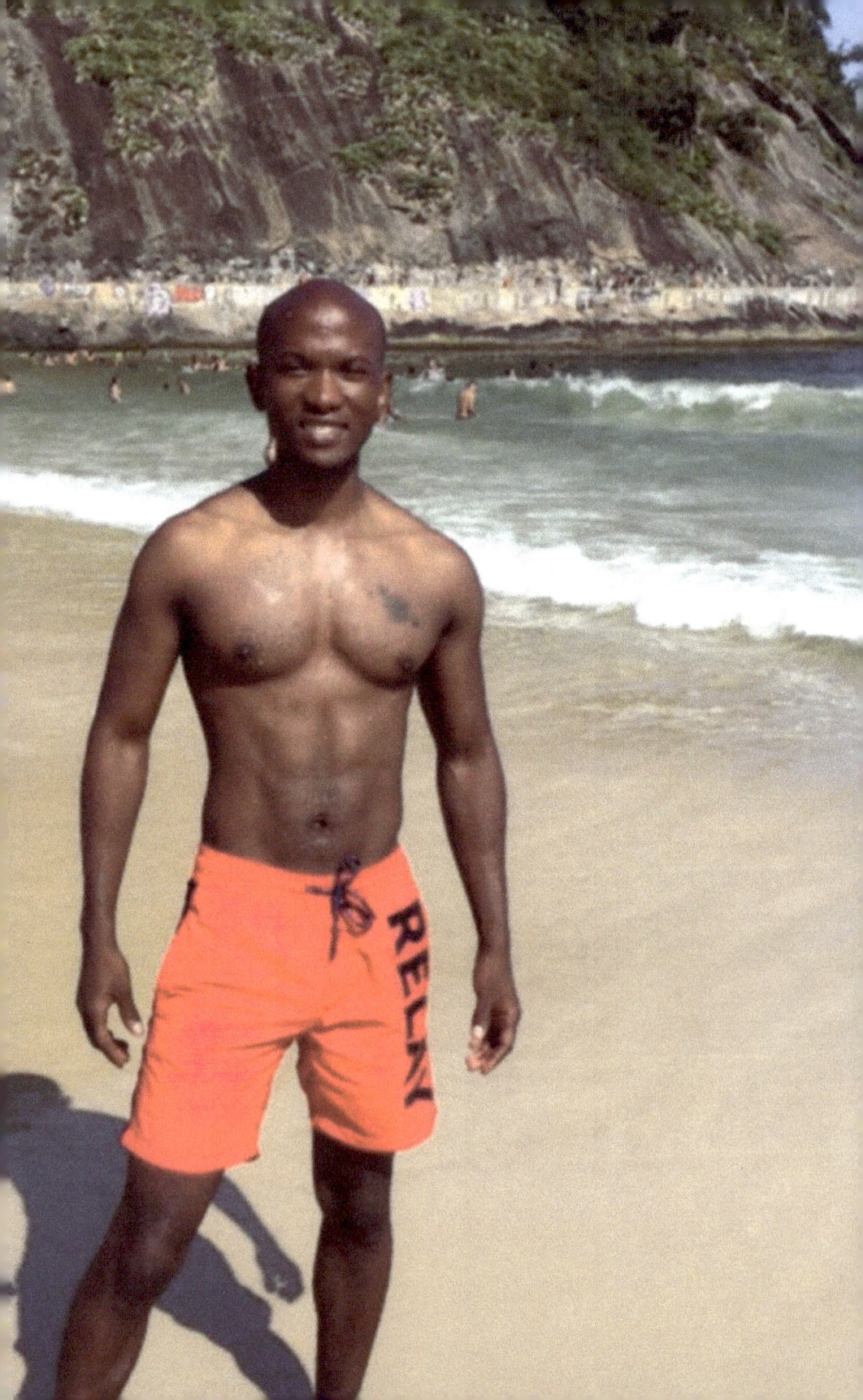

MY BODY
TRANSFORMATION STORY

My body transformation journey started when I was in high school. Little did I know this journey would turn into my passion and I would become a Personal Trainer helping people like you transform their bodies, habits, and lifestyles to be fit and healthy and have a good quality of life.

At the time, I was happy with my body, but then I changed schools. At my new school, doing a sport was compulsory. Even though I really love adventure sport - skiing and sky diving specifically, I settled with running because this was what was available. But running opened the door to a series of unexpected challenges.

After some time on the running team, I began to notice that I was losing body fat and muscle. I was not happy with the way I looked. I was getting fitter, but I did not look like an athlete. One of the problems I realised was that I was not fuelling my body correctly for running. I was not eating the right foods, and as a result, I kept losing weight and muscle tone.

I started losing self-confidence and developed a negative self-perception.

One day, after feeling really down, I told myself – " Sizwe, you can either stay this way, OR you can do something about it."

I decided that I was going to do something!

I figured that by joining a gym, I could change my body image and regain my self-confidence.

I visited the gym close by and approached a sales consultant. I discussed my reasons for joining the gym.

"You have come to the right place," the consultant reassured me. "We have a fitness team here that will help you to achieve your goals."

I was relieved. I had found a solution; I was on my way!

I imagined that joining the gym was going to solve my problems, but I was about to find a whole new set of obstacles and challenges.

I'm sure my story will sound familiar to you.

As a student, with no income at the time, I convinced my parents to pay for my gym membership. Luckily, they agreed. I signed up and was the proud owner of a membership card that allowed me into the gym whenever I wanted. I was excited!

On my first day at the gym, I arrived all pumped up, motivated, and ready to start. I could even see my ideal body - my chest muscles, my biceps – a six-pack!

I looked around for the sales consultant who had signed me up, thinking he would be there to assist me. But the consultant was nowhere to be seen.

I went back to the receptionist. I explained that this was my first day and I needed assistance. She smiled and arranged for a floor assistant to show me around the gym.

The floor assistant showed me the cardio machines as fast as he could. He showed me the steam rooms and other facilities I didn't need for my body transformation goals. And then, he disappeared.

I expected a bit more interest from the gym staff. I realised very quickly that a gym membership really means that I was renting the use of the machines, nothing more.

I used the machines the floor assistant showed me for a while before I realised that I wasn't seeing any results. I felt like this was a waste of time. I was not moving any closer to my goals.

My start at the gym was disappointing. I felt despondent. On top of this, my muscles were painful after my workouts. I definitely wasn't enjoying this! But I continued because I was determined to achieve my goals.

I felt like giving up many days, but somehow, I had to dig deep and managed to carry on going to the gym.

My parents agreed to pay for a Personal Trainer because I could see that I needed someone to help me understand what I needed to do to reach my goals. But finding the right Trainer proved to be another challenge.

There were two Personal Trainers at my gym. I spoke to the male trainer first. He was muscular, and I thought he would be the right person to help me. But it turned out that he was unfriendly and didn't really show real interest in me.

I then approached the second trainer. She was friendly and listened to me. She took the time to show me resistance exercises. She explained different types of resistance training. I began to understand how resistance training could help me to build muscle. I felt motivated again. With her to guide me, I began to believe that I would be able to reach my goals again.

She taught me about nutrition, then gave me an eating plan - free of charge! The eating plan was what I needed to support my goals.

I started to realise that body transformation is more than just exercising; it is about the right nutrition too.

One of the changes I had to make was preparing my own meals at home. Instead of eating family meals, I needed different meals based on the advice from my Personal Trainer. This took a lot of effort and planning.

So now, I had a Personal Trainer, an exercise programme, and a nutrition plan. I felt more confident that I was getting somewhere. This was great! I started feeling motivated.

As my training progressed, I found that my personal trainer was also my first point of support. She motivated me and gave me feedback on my progress. This made me realise how important it is to have people around me who would be supportive.

I also realised that if I wanted to be successful, I needed to be focused on my goal both inside and outside the gym. I needed a lifestyle that was in line with my goals.

My social life began to change. My friends at the time were not very supportive of my new lifestyle. For example, I started using my pocket money to buy protein and vitamin supplements. My friends found this strange. In the end, I began to spend less and less time with them. I didn't find going out and drinking fun anymore.

I made new friends at the gym. We supported each other by buying supplements together in bulk. We also went out to eat after the gym which made it easier to choose healthy meals because I was among friends who chose to eat the same way I did. This really helped me to speed up my results. Whenever I wasn't at the gym, I would get a text message from my new friends to find out why I missed training.

Once I started getting fit, I focused on pushing myself as hard as I could in training. I wanted to see results. Resting after a workout was something that I neglected. My personal trainer didn't emphasise the importance of rest either.

I became so addicted to training that even when I went on holiday, whether it was a local or an international trip, I would look for a gym so I could work out.

I became addicted to muscle pump. This is done for optimal for muscle growth. The pump is when your muscles swell up during your workout and is caused by an excessive amount of blood going into the muscle and filling it up the same way you would fill up a water balloon.

During this time, I developed mild shoulder joint pain. I ignored the pain. I was starting to see results and pushed through the pain.

When I introduced rest days into my training, the pain in my shoulders went away completely. I am now pain-free.

After two years of being at the gym, I felt like a completely different person. I was happier with my body and my image and was starting to feel more confident within myself.

When I reached my body transformation goal, my choice of clothes started changing. I could wear anything I wanted to. I wore more sleeveless shirts and vests and other clothes. I could take off my shirt and sit by the pool and wear shorts- even though I couldn't swim.

I was proud of my body and the hard work I had put in.

I had more energy, and I started to enjoy physical work. Whenever there were heavy things that needed to be moved at home, I was called to do it.

"Ask Sizwe to move that; he is the strong one."

I guess this was a way to pay my parents back for covering my gym fees!

But my step into fully into the world of health and fitness was still ahead.

After high school, I began studying towards a degree in Marketing and Business Management.

During the first year, I became one of the popular students because of my self-confidence. I passed my first year.

In my second year, I was approached to enter a competition at my colleges. Before developing confidence through my training and body transformation, this was something that I would never have considered doing. I entered and made the top five!

After the competition, I looked back at what had gotten me there. I realised that training at the gym with a Personal Trainer was the reason I had changed. I felt inspired to become a Personal Trainer, realising that I wanted to share this experience and to help other people go through the transformation I did. This was what I wanted to do with my life. It was at this point that I set as my life's goal to help people who were in a similar position that I had been in.

Before the new year started, I changed my marketing and business management studies to a Personal Training course.

The day I completed my Personal Training course was the day that a whole new journey began for me.

During my early days of being a Personal Trainer, one of my colleague, a friend and mentor to me, and an experienced Personal Trainer told me that even though I looked great, my posture could be improved. I had mainly focused on training my chest and front muscles, which is what one sees when standing in front of the mirror. I had neglected my back muscles, which resulted in me having a rounded spine.

I started researching exercises for posture correction - and this is how I discovered yoga. I studied Satyananda yoga, based on Swami Satyananda teachings.

Over time, I grew to love a yoga meditation technique- Yoga Nidra.

The main benefit of this practice is developing awareness.

I believe that by practising this technique, you can become aware of your unique gifts. It definitely helped me to find mine. My mantra is: "I love life." And I do!

But there was much more I was going to learn through yoga.

After practising yoga for a few months, I started noticing physical and emotional differences. I realised that I no longer was short-tempered and aggressive; I realised that I was calmer, more patient, and relaxed.

My posture had improved, and once again, I was happy to have reached another goal.

I started teaching yoga to groups of people.

Over the years, I have spent a lot of time evolving my personal fitness practice. The result is the book you are holding in your hand.

My specialisation is training both males and females over the age of 45; helping them to develop stress management techniques, stay fit as they age, have less or no musculoskeletal pain, have good quality sleep, improve their quality of life, and feel great about themselves.

I share my story with you, hoping that it will inspire you to overcome your challenges, whatever they are, and begin or continue your journey to being your best self.

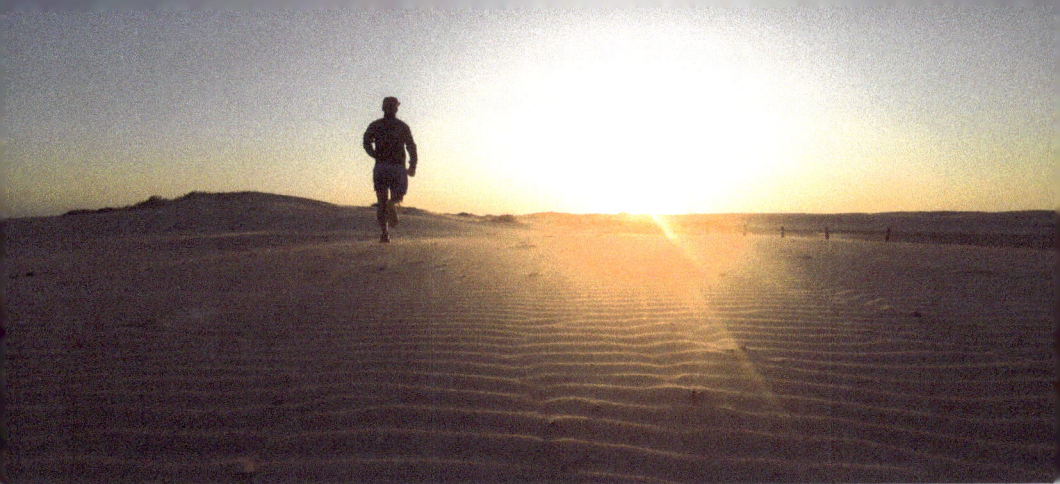

CHAPTER 1
GETTING STARTED

"If you don't know where you're going, any road can take you there."
Lewis Carroll

We would all like to have a great body, feel confident about ourselves, be fit, and have a great quality of life. But how do we achieve this?

The first step is to have a clear idea of your starting point. You need to know exactly where you are with your health and fitness so that you can plan for where you would like to be.

Creating a starting point will help you have a realistic sense of your fitness level, weight, and how much you want to gain or lose to plan for the kind of body and the fitness level you want to have. Get to know your own body and how it works before you can start to transform it in a way that suits you.

What do I need to create a starting point?
You need to do three things to discover your starting point.

First, you need to know if you are healthy enough to start a body transformation plan. You have to know about any health challenges like high or low blood pressure and how to manage this so that you can participate in a programme. The best way to do this is to have yourself checked out by a Doctor.

Second, you need to assess your body by weighing and measuring yourself through a comprehensive body composition assessment. You can do this yourself, with a friend, or with a Personal Trainer.

Third, you need to do a fitness assessment. A fitness assessment identifies your current fitness level, which will help to decide what exercise goals you need to set. You can then track your progress over time.

Following these three steps will help you discover your body transformation starting point.

Keeping weekly and monthly, even daily records of how you are doing will let you know if you are on track to reach your body transformation goals.

But how will I know how to do all of this?
I have set each of these three steps out in detail in this chapter. So, you don't have to worry about anything.

If you have a Personal Trainer, they will take you through these steps on your first day.

STEP 1: AM I HEALTHY ENOUGH TO PARTICIPATE IN A BODY TRANSFORMATION PLAN?
The first, most important step is to consult your doctor before you start any exercise and eating programme.

If you decide to work with a Personal Trainer, they will ask you these questions and keep a record of your health status and develop a safe exercise plan, especially for you.

HEALTH QUESTIONNAIRE

- Has your doctor indicated that you have a heart condition? Yes/No
  If yes, describe your heart condition

- Has your doctor ever said that your blood pressure was too high or low? Yes/No
  If yes, describe your condition.

- Do you have any bone, back, or other joint conditions that may be aggravated by exercise? Yes/No.
  If yes, describe your condition.

- Do you suffer from epilepsy or asthma? Yes/No
  If yes, describe your condition

Do you suffer from diabetes? Yes/No

Are you pregnant? Yes/No

- Are you taking any prescribed medication that may affect your ability to exercise? Yes/No
  If yes, list the medication you are taking

- Do you smoke? Yes/No
  If yes, describe your smoking habits

```


```

- Are there any other reasons why exercise is not suitable for you?
  Describe this.

```


```

Why Is Knowing All This Information Important?
Knowing your health status means that you can exercise safely and will ensure that you are not harming your body in any way.

Whatever your condition, share it with your Personal Trainer. They will consider your health when designing a programme for you.

Remember that you are unique. All this information will help you to know your body and your health.

STEP 2: BODY COMPOSITION ASSESSMENT AND MEASUREMENTS

What is body composition, and why should I know about it?
Body composition describes the percentages of fat, bone, water, and muscle in human bodies. A healthy balance between fat and muscle is vital for health and wellness throughout life.

What is the benefit of having a good body composition?
Healthy body composition will increase your lifespan; reduce the risk of heart disease, cancer, diabetes, and insulin resistance. It will also increase energy levels.

So now that you know whether you are healthy enough to participate in a body transformation programme, the next thing you need is a comprehensive body composition assessment.

A Personal Trainer will do an assessment with you, or you can do this by yourself or ask a friend to help you.

There are 14 areas you are going to measure, assess, and record to discover your starting point.

You will need a tape measure, a body scanning scale, and a blood pressure machine.

With your measuring tape, you are going to measure your height, waist, hip, chest, upper arm, upper leg, and calves.

Your body-scanning scale will give you your weight, body mass index (BMI), body fat percentage, water percentage, bone mineral content.

Finally, your blood pressure machine will give you a reading of your blood pressure.

Assessment Sheet

Your personal trainer will use this sheet or a similar one to record your progress.

Date				
Height				
Weight				
Body Mass Index (BMI)				
Waist				
Hip				
Chest				
Upper Arm				
Upper Leg				
Calves				
Body Fat %				
Blood Pressure				
Resting Heart Rate				
Water %				
Muscle				
Bone				

Why are these fourteen areas essential, and what do these readings mean?

Body Measurements

Taking accurate body measurements is important for tracking your weight and centimetres loss or gain accurately.

Tips About Measuring

- You need to use a soft tape measure, one that curves around your body easily.

- When measuring, do not pull the tape too tightly. Keep it just level across your skin.

Measuring Your Height
- Stand bare feet with your feet flat on the floor and your heels against the wall.
- Make sure your head, shoulders, and buttocks are touching the wall.
- Stand up straight. Your line of sight and chin should be parallel to the floor.
- Take your measurement right against your head.

Waist Measurements
Place the tape around the belly button part of your waist; remember to always place the tape measure over the same part of your body every time you measure to get an accurate reading.

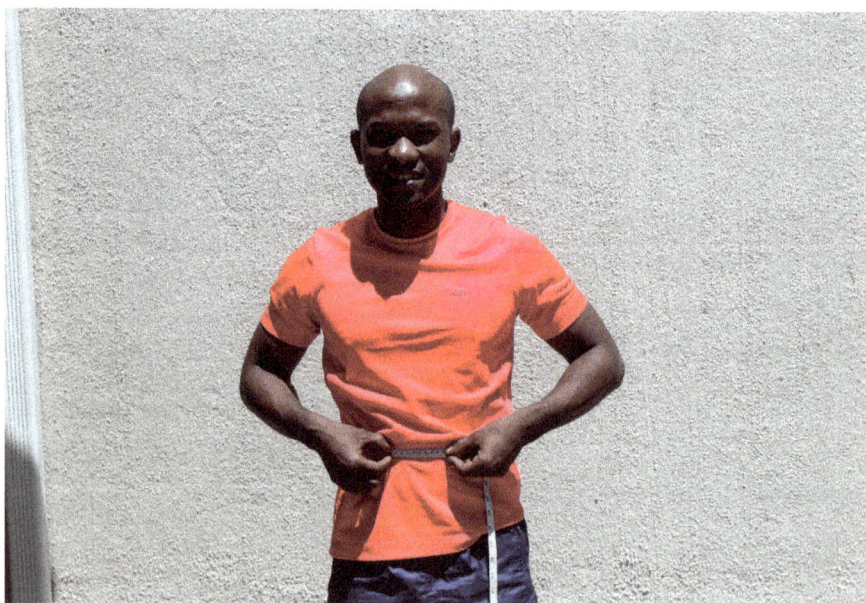

- Female's waist measurement needs to be 83 cm. It is a health risk when it exceeds 88 cm.
- Male's waist measurements need to be 88 cm. It is a health risk when it exceeds 103 cm.

Arm Measurements
- Place the tape around the middle of the top of your arm.

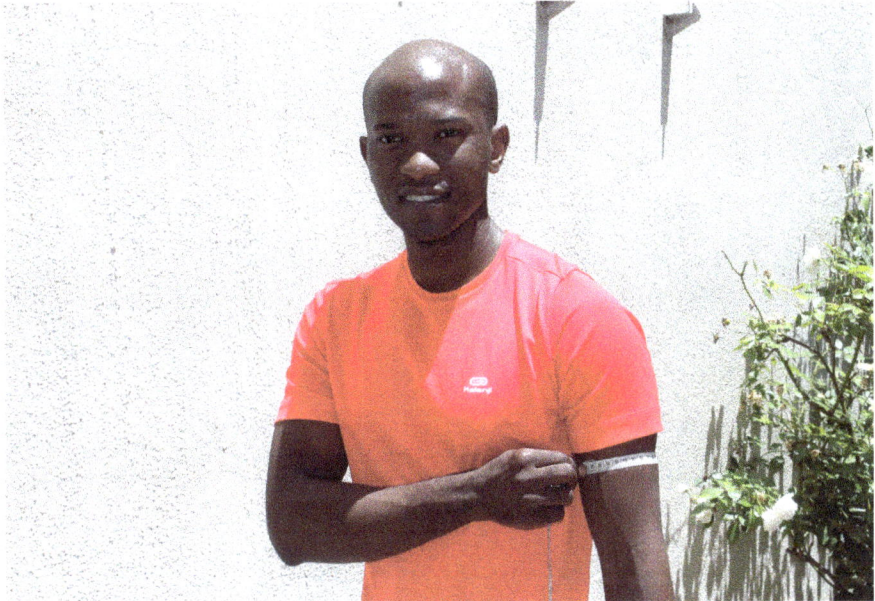

Calves

- Place the tape so that you measure the widest section of your calf.

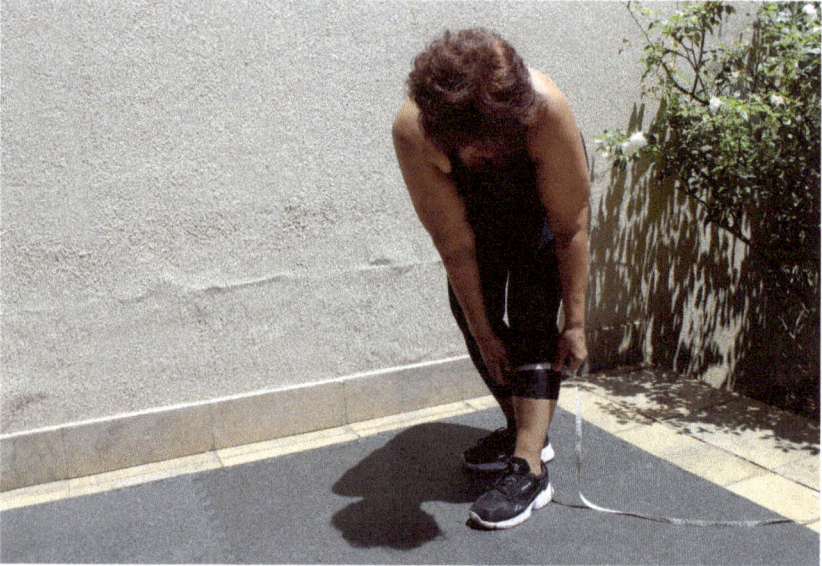

Thighs

- Place the tape around the middle section of your thigh.

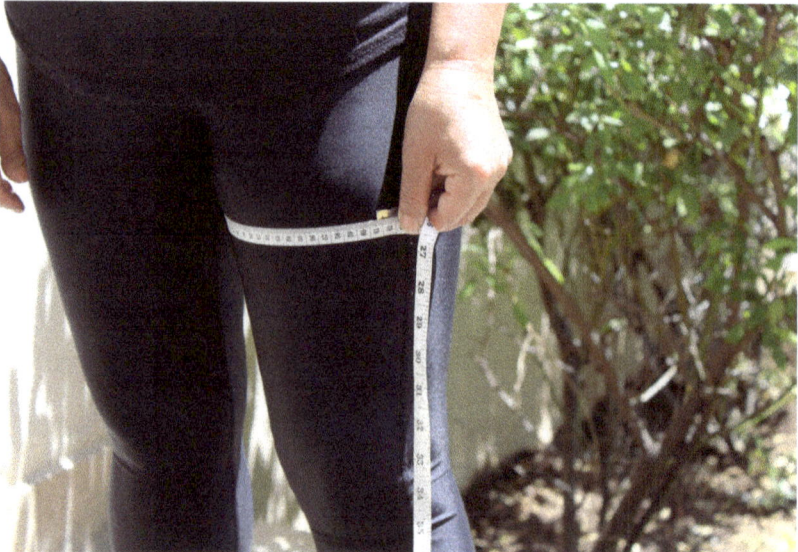

Hip

- Position the tape around the widest part of the buttock.

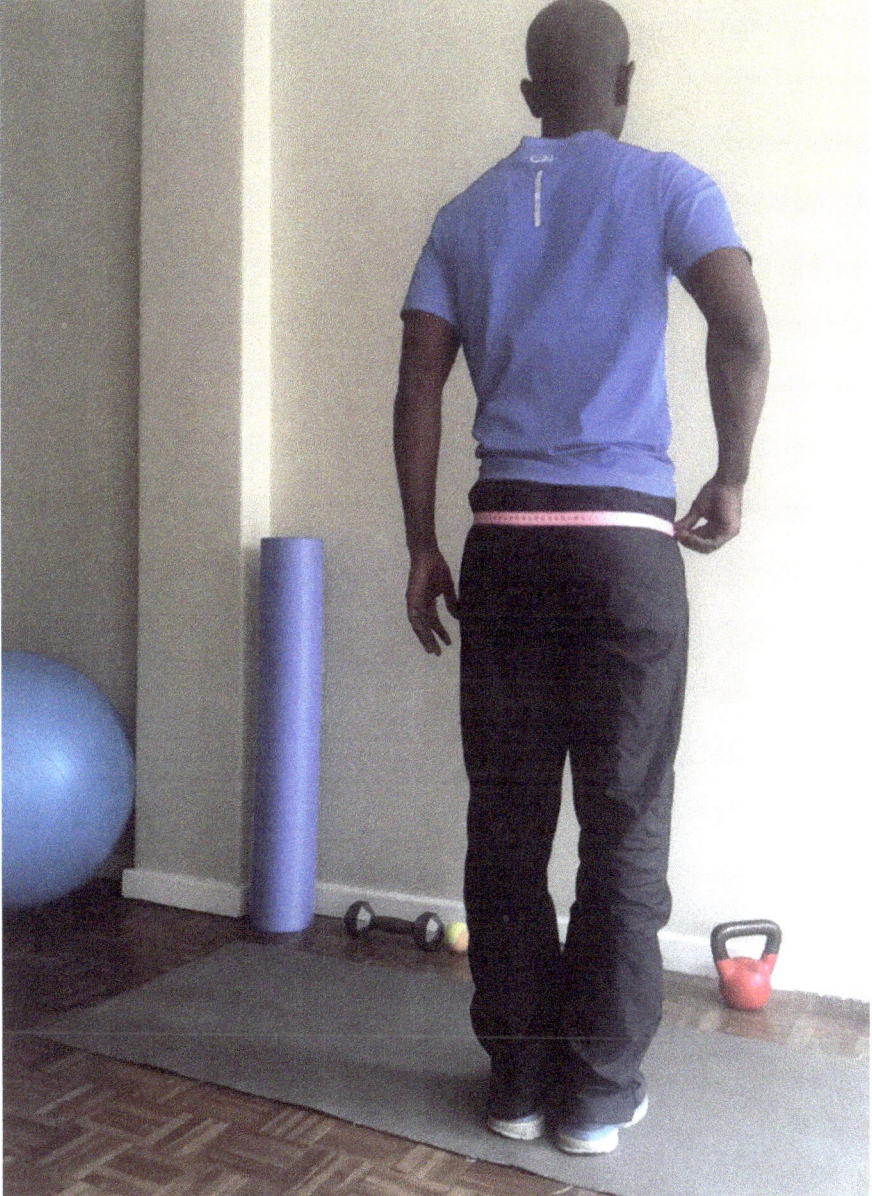

Chest

- Position the tape on top of the nipples.
- For women, wear the same bra every time you measure to get an accurate reading.

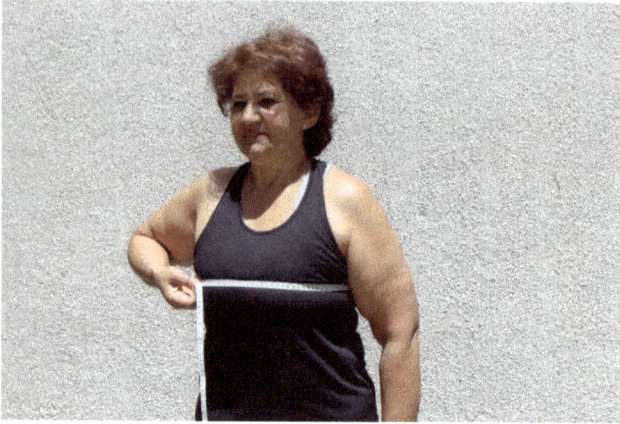

For the next set of measurements, you will need a body-scanning scale.

Weight

Tracking weight loss on a scale will show that weight loss is not always constant. When you exercise, you are building muscle, which can lead to weight gain. Muscle weighs more than fat, so what can seem like weight gain (or fat gain) on a scale may actually just be muscle gain.

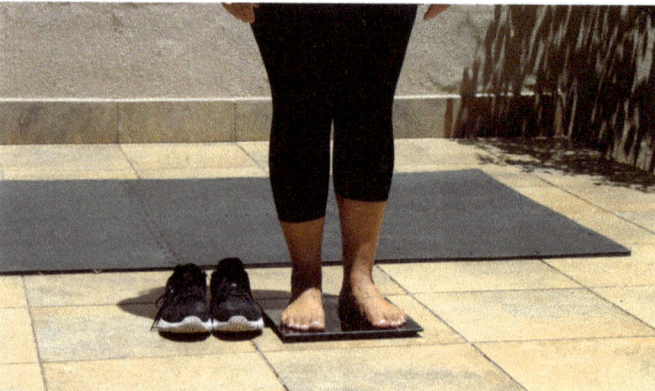

- The best time to weigh yourself is in the morning after you have been to the loo, wearing as little clothing as possible.
- Place your scale on a hard, even surface, not on carpeting.
- Stand still with your weight distributed evenly on both feet.

Body Mass Index (BMI)

Body mass index (BMI) is a measure of your body fat based on your height and weight. It is a measure that tells you if your weight is healthy.

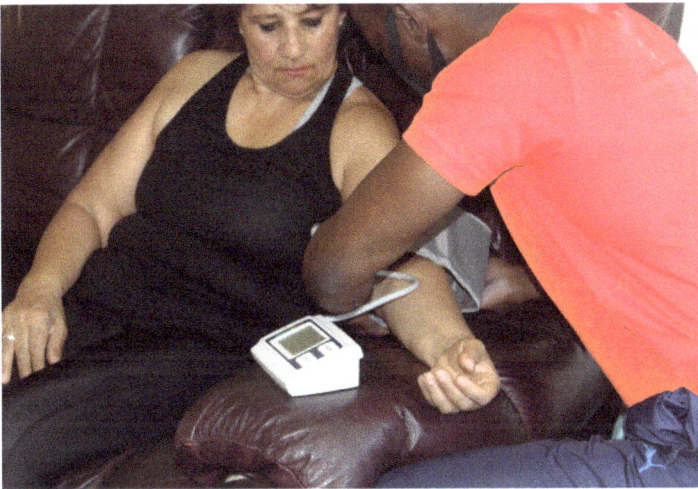

This formula calculates your BMI

Height(m) x Height(M)/ Weight(kg) = BMI

Example: My height is 1.69cm, and my weight is 60kgs
Using the formula, this is how I calculate my BMI:
1.69 x 1.69 = 2.8561
60kgs / 2.8561 = 21.00
My BMI is 21.00

If your BMI is

- Less than 18.5 – you're in the underweight range
- Between 18.5 and 24.9 – you're in the healthy or normal weight range
- Between 25 and 29.9 – you're in the overweight range
- Between 30 and 35 – you're in the Grade 1 obesity range (moderate risk)
- Between 35 and 40 - you're in the Grade 2 obesity range (high risk)
- Greater than 40 – you're in the Grade 3 obesity range (morbid obesity)

For most adults, an ideal BMI is in the 18.5 to 24.9 range.

Measuring your Body Fat Percentage (BFP)

Body fat percentage is a measurement of body composition that tells you how much of your body's weight is fat. The normal ranges for body fat differ for men and women.

There are different ways to measure body fat percentage, but the most common ways are using the body composition scale and a skinfold.

Using a Body Scanning Scale

- By simply stepping on the scale, you will get a reading for both your body weight and your estimated body fat percentage.

Another way to measure body fat is by doing a skinfold test.

Skinfold

- A skinfold test is done by taking a pinch of skin with callipers to determine the fat layer thickness at several points on the body.

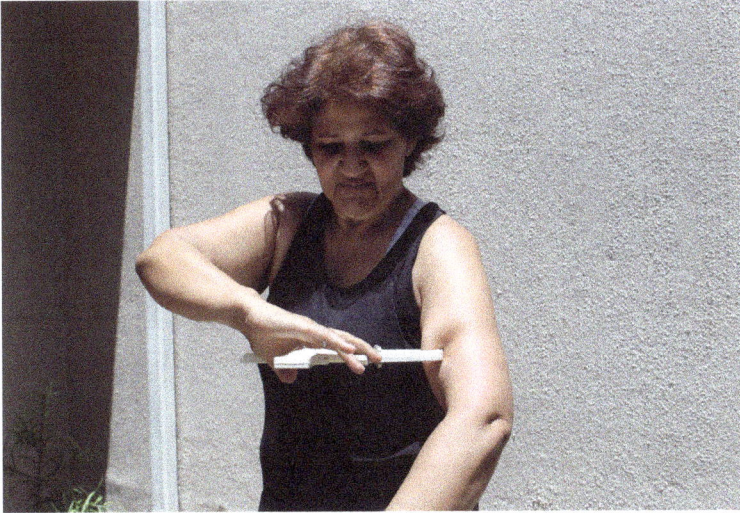

Tips for Measuring Body Fat Percentage

- It is best is to stick to one method of measuring as a different method may give you a different reading.
- It's also best to use the method that you have access to. So, if you have a body-scanning scale, stick to measuring your body fat percentage on your scale.

Guidelines for Body Fat Percentage for women and men

Description	Women	Men
Essential Fat	12-15%	2-5%
Athletes	16-20%	6-13%
Fitness	21-24%	14-17%
Acceptable	25-31%	18-25%
Overweight	32%	25%

Body Water Percentage (BWP)
The Body Water Percentage shows how hydrated your body is.

Your water composition is the percentage of body fluid as compared to total body weight.

The easiest way to measure your hydration is by using a body-scanning scale.
- The ideal percentage for adult women is between 45 and 60%.
- The ideal percentage for adult men is between 50 and 65%

Bone Mass (BM)
Bones play many roles in the body — providing structure, protecting organs, anchoring muscles, and storing calcium. By knowing your bone mass, you will know how diet, physical activity, and other lifestyle factors affect you.

- The average bone content for adults is 3-5%, and your scale will give you a reading.

Blood Pressure (BP)
Blood pressure is a measure of how hard your heart has to pump to deliver blood to all parts of your body. Without blood pressure, your body wouldn't get the oxygen it needs to survive.

The two most important measures are whether your blood pressure is too high or too low.

How to take your Blood Pressure
- Always use the same arm when taking your blood pressure.
- Rest your arm, raised to the level of your heart, on a table, desk, or chair arm. You might need to place a pillow or cushion under your arm to elevate it high enough.
- Place the cuff on bare skin, not over clothing.

Estimated Normal Blood Pressure for Different Ages

Age	Normal Systolic Range	Normal Diastolic Range
Adolescent (14–18 years)	90–120 mm Hg	50–80 mm Hg
Adult (19–40 years)	95–135 mm Hg	60–80 mm Hg
Adult (41–60 years)	110–145 mm Hg	70–90 mm Hg
Older adult (61 and older)	95–145 mm Hg	70–90 mm Hg

Now that you have completed the health, measurement, and assessments, you should have a good idea of where you are. You have one last step - a fitness test.

STEP 3 FITNESS TEST

A fitness test is an assessment of your strength, endurance, and flexibility. This assessment will help you to track the progress you are making towards becoming fit in these areas.

There are many fitness tests. This one is a mini fitness test to get you started.

Test 1: Sit and Reach
- Reach forward as far as you can; try to touch your toes.
- Be cautious if you have back problems.

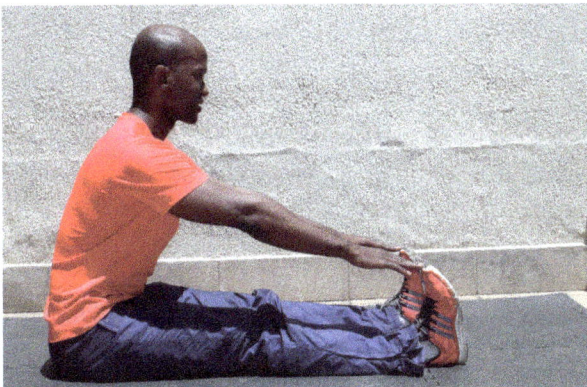

Record how far you can reach by ticking the relevant block

Date	Heels Very Good	Toes Good	Ankles Average	Shins Poor	Knees Very Poor

Test 2: Push Up Test

The correct way to do a standard push-up is to position your hands shoulder-width apart or a little bit wider.

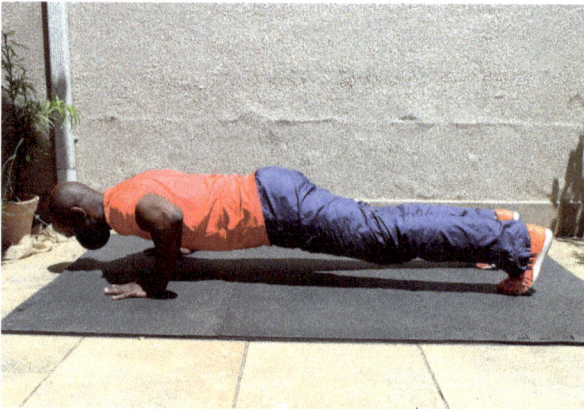

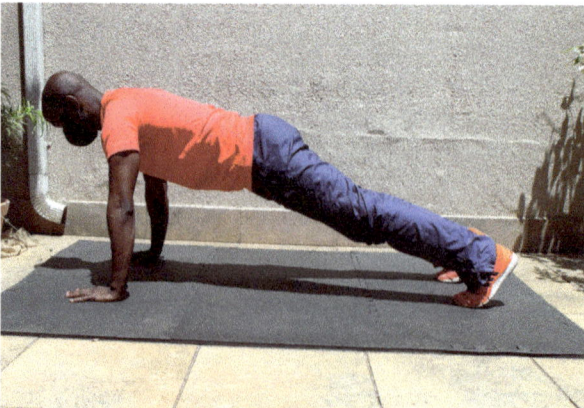

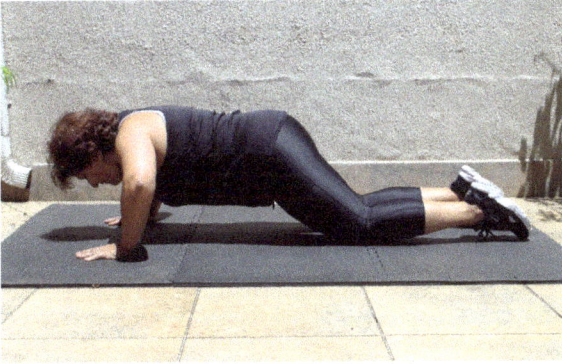

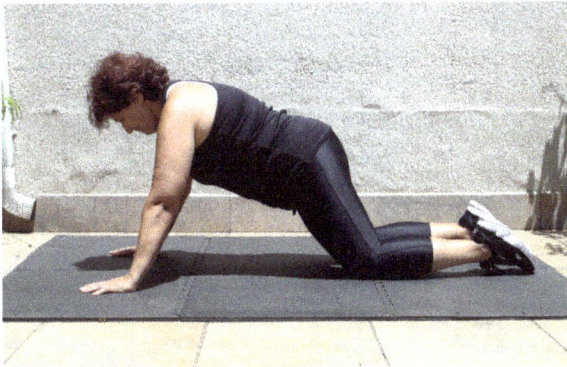

- As you bend your elbows and lower your body toward the ground, your elbows should be at about a 45-degree angle to your body,
- Men should balance on their hands and feet. Ladies should balance on their hands and knees.
- Do as many standard push-ups as you can and record the number.

Results	Females	Males
Excellent	31+	50+
Very Good	25-30	40-49
Good	13-24	31-39
Average	7-12	21-30
Poor	0-6	0-20

Test 3: Static Muscle Endurance Test – Wall Chair

- Stand with your back and shoulders flat against the wall, facing forward.
- Slide down the wall until you are in a sitting position.
- Hold this position for as long as you can, and time yourself.
- Record your time.

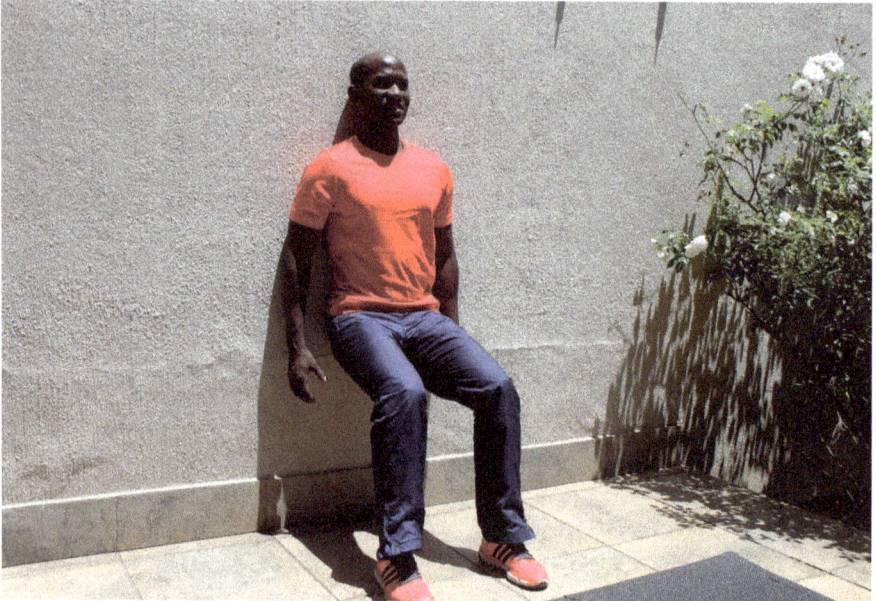

Excellent	120+ seconds
Very Good	90 -120 seconds
Good	60-90 seconds
Average	30-60 seconds
Poor	30

What Do I Do Now That I Have Completed The Assessment Measurement And Fitness Test?

Have a look over each result and think about what it is telling you.

If you have done this assessment with your Personal Trainer, they will discuss your results with you. Ask as many questions about the assessment so that you understand what they mean.

Try not to be discouraged by your results. Treat it as information and feedback to motivate you to make changes.

With the information you have, you can now decide what your health and fitness goals should be.

SETTING HEALTH AND FITNESS GOALS

By setting goals, you are setting a target to aim for. Without goals, you will not be able to manage progress.

But setting goals also takes practice. At first, you may set your goals too high or too low. If you set your goal too low, and you may find that you may not feel motivated enough. If you aim too high, you may be setting yourself up for disappointment and give up. With practice, you will set them – "just right!"

Don't be afraid to adjust your goals. Your Personal Trainer will support you all the way.

How Do I Set A Goal?

The best way to set goals is to set SMART goals - Specific, Measurable, Achievable, Realistic, and Time-Bound.

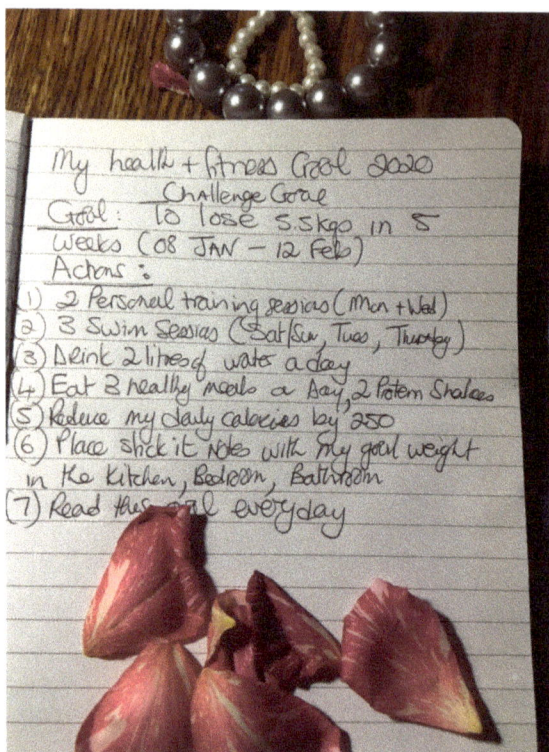

But what does this mean for health and fitness goals?

S = Specific: a goal has to be specific." I want to be fit" is not specific. A specific goal could be "I want to build up my strength so that I can hold a three-minute plank."

M – Measurable: a goal has to be measurable; otherwise, you won't know that you have achieved it. If you say: "I want to lose weight," you won't be able to say how much weight you lost. But if you say, "I want to lose 5kgs", you will know whether you are moving closer to achieving your goal every time you get onto the scale.

A = Achievable: a goal must be achievable; in other words, it must be possible to reach your goal. If you set yourself a goal like: " I want to run 10kms in 1hour in a week," if you have never run before, you will be unable to achieve this goal because it's simply unachievable. But with the right training, over time, and commitment, you can achieve this goal.

R = Realistic: A realistic goal is one that you believe can be accomplished with the time and resources you have available. We know that three minutes seems like a lifetime when you're holding a plank, but if you start slowly, 20 to 30-seconds daily, and each week, increase by 20 to 30 seconds, after about six weeks, you should be able to hold a three-minute plank.

T= Timebound: When you have a timeline - a start and end date to reach your goal, you are creating a sense of purpose and urgency to reach your goals.

So now it's time to write down your goals.
Your Personal Trainer will go through your assessments with you, or you will do it on your own. Write down the three health and fitness goals you would like to achieve.

Write down your three health and fitness goals using the SMART method. It doesn't have to be perfect. Think about the benefits of reaching this goal?

Goal 1
Goal 2
Goal 3

Have a plan for when you will exercise and commit to them.

What is the most realistic time of the day to do your activities?

How many times a week can you participate in your activities?

Taking Action!

If you want to guarantee that you will reach your goals, you have to act!

But which actions should you take?

Action 1: Write Down Your Goals –Writing down your goals will make them real. Read them every day so that they are top of mind for you.

Action 2: Identify your motivator: Understand your "Why." Find a BIG enough reason to achieve your goals so that you feel challenged and motivated.

Action 3: Develop A Plan: Write down what you need to do, what resources - equipment, even the time you need, who can support you, and anything else you need to achieve your goals.

Action 4: Set A Deadline: By when do you want to achieve your goals? Create some urgency for yourself; use a special milestone or event to motivate you, like a sports event or a special family occasion.

Action 5: Start! Don't say, "I'll start Monday or next week." Start the right way! Start anywhere. But start.

Well done on getting this far! You have discovered your starting point, and you have set your goals.

In the next chapters, you will find out what the five body transformation codes are and how they can help you meet your goals.

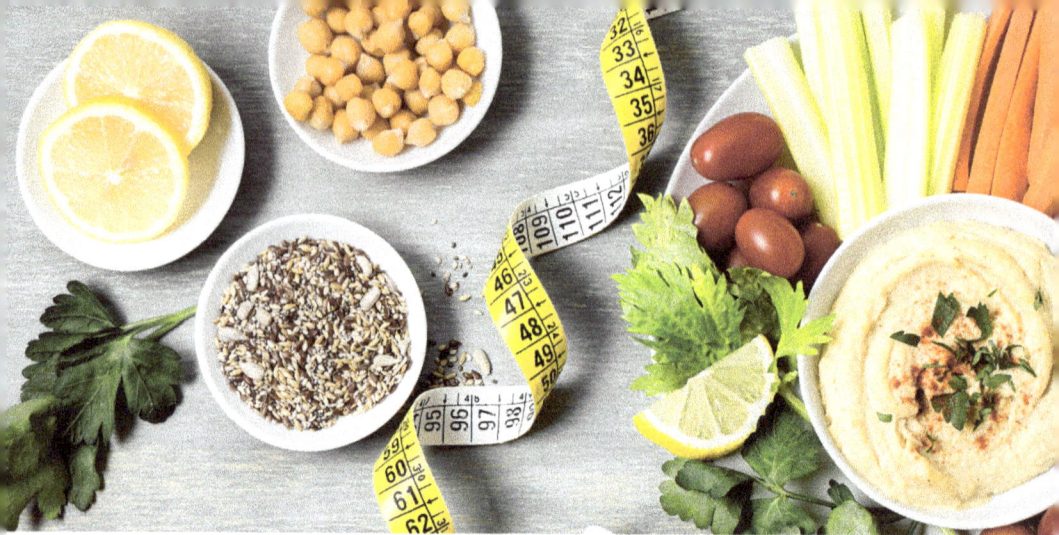

CHAPTER 2
CODES FOR GREAT NUTRITION AND HYDRATION

"Healthy does NOT mean starving yourself EVER. Healthy means eating the right food in the right amount."
=Karen Salmansohn

Have you decided what you want your body to look like? If you haven't, don't carry on reading.
Stop!

Close your eyes, visualise, have a look at some pictures, imagine your ideal body. Do you want to lose weight? Or gain weight? Or are you trying to build muscle? Don't continue until you have made your decision.

Many everyday gadgets help us to function in our lives. Think about it, your car, your GPS, your watch, each of these gadgets has a special computer coding that tells the computer inside it what to do so that it does what it is supposed to do.

In a similar way, our bodies need codes to transform them – if we want to build muscle, we need to code our bodies in a certain way so that it can perform the task of building muscle.

In this chapter, I'm going to tell you about the 20% nutrition and hydration codes you need to know for your body transformation goals.

There are many nutrition and hydration codes, but to start with, I'm going to explain five of these: (1) Eating high-quality food, (2) How frequently you should eat, (3) Macronutrients, (4) Calorie intake, and (5) Hydration.

Why Are Nutrition and Hydration the First Code?

We are what we eat and drink
We all have to eat every day; this is why good food and drink choices are the first code for body transformation.

The human body is an incredibly diverse organism made up of billions of cells that operate in different ways, and each need different nutrients at different times to operate at an optimum level.

This is why the food choices you make every single meal or snack, every single day, can make or break your journey towards your health and fitness goals.

Body transformation starts with choosing to eat in a certain way and consuming the right food for you to be able to change your body image and look great. Nutrition and hydration may form only 20% of 100%, but it is a very important 20%.

Why is Food so important?

Nutrition is at the centre of transforming your body – whether you are trying to shed fat, gain weight, or build muscle. Good nutrition will support your body to operate at an optimum level so that it can be transformed into what you want.

Some signs will tell you that your body is not functioning optimally – you will feel fatigued, your toilet habits change, and you generally don't feel energised. You need an eating plan that is structured, consistent, and designed to help achieve your goals. There are no two ways about this.

A good eating plan will provide nutrients for things like energy for activity, growth, and other functions of the body, such as breathing, digesting food and keeping warm. Good nutrition provides materials for the growth and repair of the body and keeping your immune system healthy.

What we choose to eat will affect what our bodies look like and how they perform during daily activities, as well as how we perform during an exercise programme.

So now that you know why nutrition is important let's talk about the nutrition coding you need to transform your body.

The first code to transforming your body is to eat high-quality food.

What Is High-Quality Food?

High-quality foods will look good in its size, shape, colour, gloss, consistency, texture, and flavour. So, if you were shopping for high-quality foods, you would look for vegetables and fruits that are grown naturally, whole grains, healthy fats, and healthy sources of protein such as free-range or organic chicken.

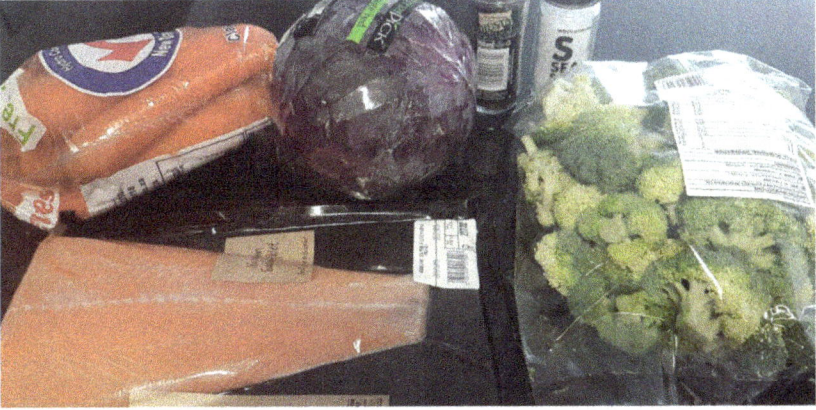

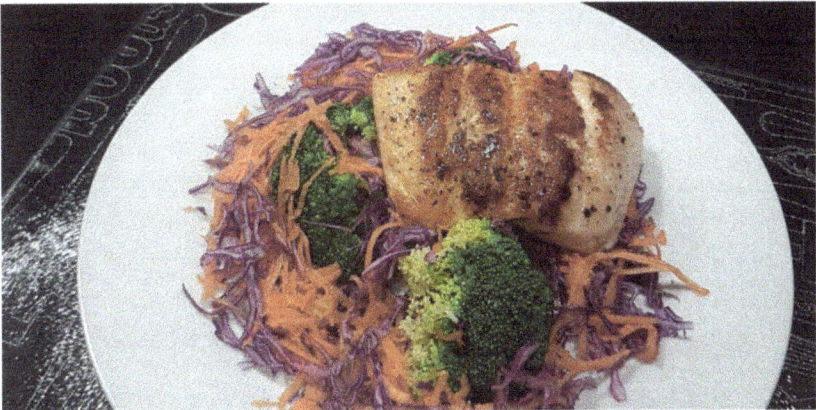

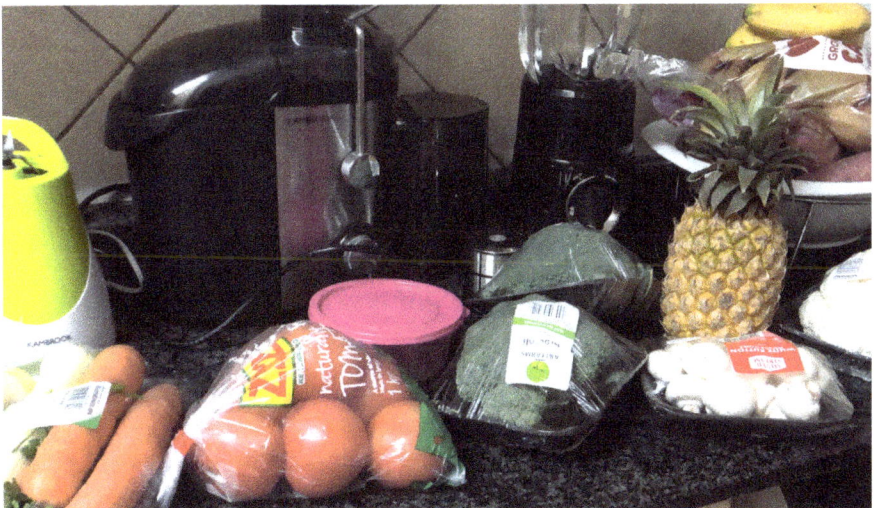

Are High-Quality Foods Easy to Find?
Often when shopping, the food in your local supermarket may not tick every box for high-quality food. But the more you become aware of what high-quality food is, the easier it will become to find them and include them in your meals.

I have developed a guide you can use for choosing high-quality foods when you are shopping. This will help you to choose foods that have fewer toxins and fake ingredients.

1. Learn to read food labels so that you can understand what is in their ingredients. "Natural flavouring" may sound good, but do you know what that means? The best way to avoid being misled by product labels is to avoid processed foods altogether.

2. Locally grown and produced food is always healthier than imported foods. This is because many imported foods are picked before they are ripe and delivered weeks later. The longer fruits and vegetables have been cut off from their life source, the fewer nutrients they will contain.

3. Seasonal foods usually taste much better than those not in season. Fruits and vegetables on the shelves that are in season will be less expensive, and they are higher in nutrients than food that is grown and sold out of season.

4. Organic foods are free from any pesticides or chemicals. They have no artificial substances added and are not genetically modified. Look for a sign that says the food is organic.

These are a few ideas of where to start your search for a good or high-quality food. These guidelines are the start of a blueprint for where to begin. Once you get started, it will begin to get easier to select high-quality foods.

How Often Should I Eat?

You may not believe this, but you have to eat five to six times a day to transform your body. Yes, you read correctly, five to six times a day - breakfast, lunch, dinner, and two to three snacks in between meals and an optional snack after dinner if you feel hungry.

Eating six small meals a day instead of two or three larger ones is a weight-loss strategy that works for many people because eating more frequently may offer the benefits of decreasing hunger and means that you don't overeat at your next meal. Eating more often means that your body has more opportunities to burn calories because of the energy involved in digesting, absorbing, and metabolising nutrients in the food.

Another reason for eating more often is that when you do not support your body with enough food, your metabolism drops, and you burn fewer calories.

Meal Planning

To be successful with a five-six meal eating plan, it's helpful to do meal planning and to try to stick to a structured eating schedule. It's a good idea to plan and cook some meals in advance so that you have them ready for when you need them. If you have a busy lifestyle, you may not have time to prepare meals and may end up grabbing anything convenient to eat, which may not be healthy or even filling.

Breakfast, lunch, and dinner need to be balanced meals. A balanced

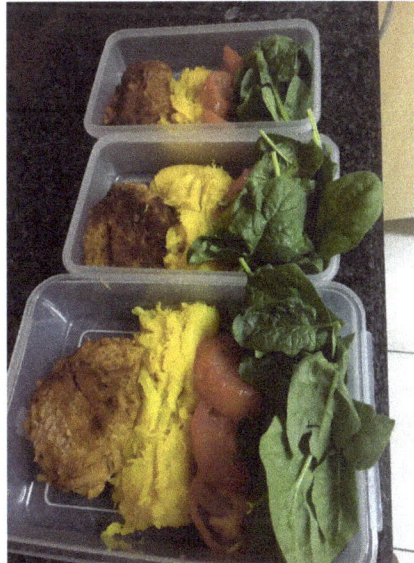

meal means paying attention to macronutrients - carbohydrates, protein, and healthy fats. Your body needs to be supported with not only enough calories to support your energy needs; it also needs the right proportions of nutrients (carbs, fats, proteins) and vitamins and minerals.

What Are Macronutrients?

Macro means large, and your body needs these three nutrients(carbs, fats, and proteins) in larger amounts to function properly.

Why Do I Need Carbohydrates To Transform my Body?

Carbs are one of the main ways the body obtains energy or calories; in fact, carbohydrates are the body's main source of energy.

Carbohydrates provide us with energy and fuel us mentally and physically. Though often spoken of negatively in some eating plans, carbohydrates are one of the basic food groups, and are important for a healthy diet.

Which Foods Contain Carbohydrates?

They are the sugars, starches, and fibres found in fruits, grains, vegetables, and milk products, vegetables, whole grain, fruits, beans, nuts, rice, and potatoes,

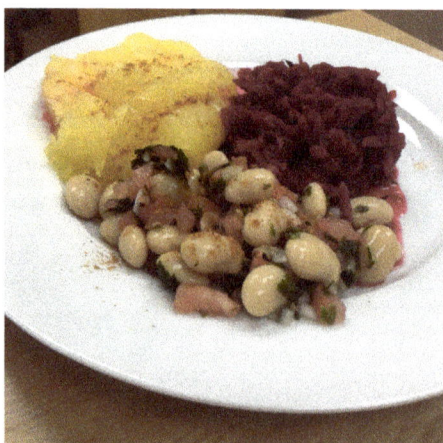

Good Carbs vs Bad Carbs

Carbohydrates that are good for you are whole grains, fruits, vegetables, beans, and legumes. These are processed more slowly in your body and keep you full for longer.

Then there are carbs you know are not good - like doughnuts, pastries, fizzy drinks, highly processed foods such as white rice and white bread.

Not having enough carbs can cause problems because, without sufficient fuel, the body will not have energy.

Why Do I Need Protein To Transform my Body?

Protein is a macronutrient that is essential to building muscle mass and burn fat. It boosts our metabolism, decreases inflammation, and helps us maintain a healthy brain and a healthy heart. Protein builds, maintains, and repairs tissue.

Which Foods Contain Protein?

Meat, poultry, seafood, beans and peas, eggs, processed soy products, nuts(almonds, cashews & other) and seeds(pumpkin, sunflower & others), yoghurt, protein bar, cheese, biltong (beef, ostrich, and others), legumes and avocado are considered part of the protein group.

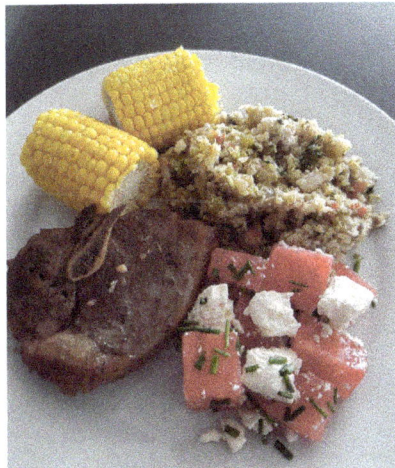

Besides animal sources, there are several alternative protein sources, including soy, hemp, and whey. All of these are good options, and really is your personal preference and your goals. For example, whey protein is the best for building and regenerating muscle mass, so you may choose whey protein if you want to bulk up or exercise regularly.

Why Do We Need Fats To Transform Our Bodies?
Fat is a nutrient, and just like protein and carbohydrates, your body needs some fat for energy, to absorb vitamins, and to protect your heart and brain health.

Although fats get a bad rap, it is an important nutrient our bodies need to function. Consuming too much fat or too little may cause health problems, so eating the right amount of fat helps to maintain good health.

Types of Fat
Saturated fats and trans fats such as milk and white chocolate, toffee, cakes, puddings and biscuits, pastries and pies, and fatty meat, such as lamb chops, processed meat sausages, burgers, and bacon, are commonly considered unhealthy.

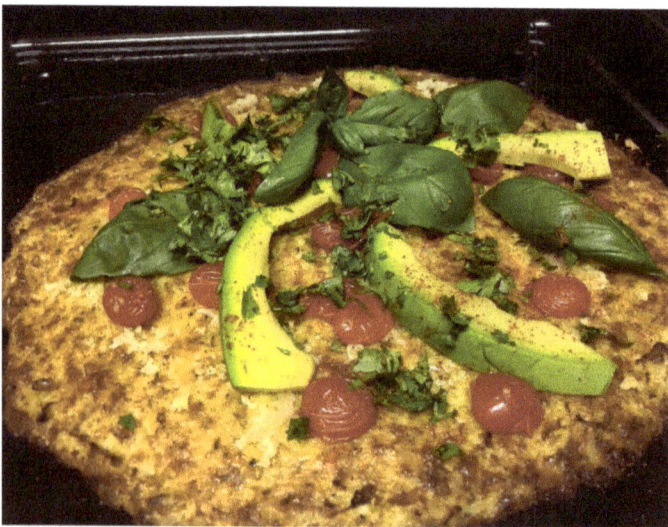

Unsaturated fats, like monounsaturated and polyunsaturated fat, are considered healthy.

Good fats to eat are avocados, cheese, dark chocolate, whole eggs, fatty fish, nuts, chia seeds, extra virgin olive oil, and full-fat yoghurt.

How to Balance Macronutrients
It is important to include each of the macronutrients in your meals every day. This will be easier if you build each meal around a combination of protein, carbs, and healthy fats. But finding the exact balance of macros, that's right for you can be tricky because everyone's body functions differently when various ratios are consumed.

The best way to track your daily macros is to use an app. There are many free apps that you can download and use.

Calorie Intake
Just as you plan your macronutrients, you need to plan your calorie intake.

A calorie is a unit of energy. When something contains 100 calories, that is a way of knowing how much energy your body could get from this food.

An ideal daily intake of calories varies depending on age, metabolism, and levels of physical activity, among other things. Generally, the recommended daily calorie intake is 2,000 calories a day for women and 2,500 for men.

What should my calorie intake be if I want to lose, maintain, or gain weight?
To be in a calorie deficit (to lose weight), the average woman needs to eat about 1,500 calories per day to lose 1/2kg a week, (on average)

and 2,000 calories per day to maintain her weight. If you need to gain weight, you need to eat more than 2,000 calories a day.

The average man needs 2,500 calories to maintain and 2,000 to lose 1/2kg per week (on average). If you want to gain weight, you need to eat more than 2,500 calories a day.

So now you know the basic codes for great nutrition. But I'm sure there is something you are dying to ask.......

What about cheat days?
And....

Do I Have To Follow The Eating Programme 100% All The Time?
NO
If you follow good eating habits 75 % of the time, you will still be able to transform your body.

When I go paragliding and skiing with friends, I eat whatever my friends are eating. Having a regular day each week to eat your favourite foods and whatever you like can be good for weight loss. It prevents binges, reduces cravings, and gives you a mental break from measuring every portion and counting calories.

I have clients who go on business lunches and eat whatever they like and still stay on track.

What Should I Do When I Eat Badly?
If you get distracted and don't follow your eating programme, even if it's for a few days, don't let it discourage you and make you think you won't be able to achieve your transformation goals. Get back and start following the programme again. Life will get you distracted now and then.

Next, I'm going to tell you about the code for staying hydrated and why this is important for body transformation.

What is Hydration, and is it important for Body Transformation?
Every system in your body depends on water so that it can perform optimally. Water is a building block to almost every cell in the body. Carbohydrates and proteins used for energy are transported by water in the bloodstream, so it helps to transport nutrients to give you energy, keep you healthy, regulate your body temperature, and lubricate your joints. If you're not properly hydrated, your body can't perform at its best.

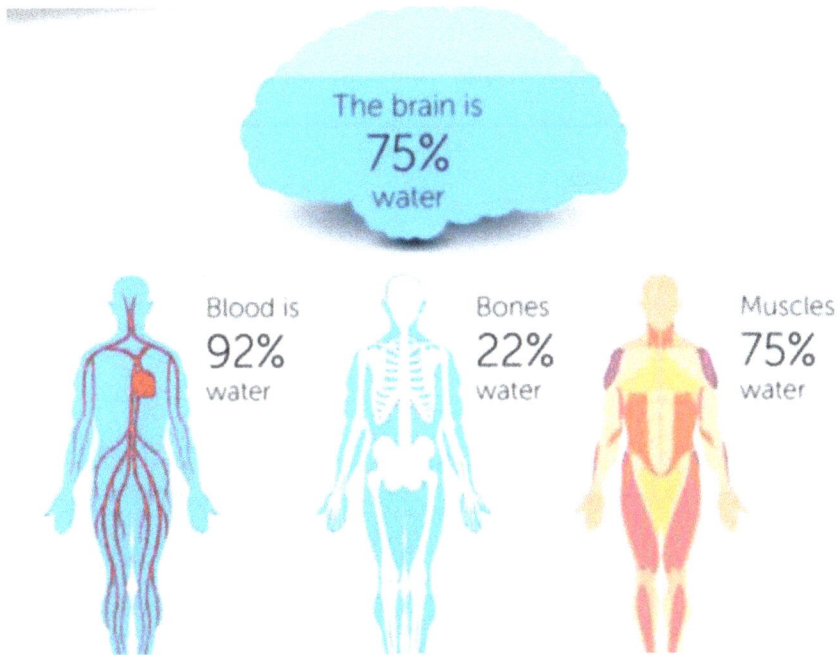

The brain is
75%
water

Blood is
92%
water

Bones
22%
water

Muscles
75%
water

To stay hydrated, you need to drink enough water and eat foods that have high water content.

Meeting your daily water intake is equally as important as eating right to stay healthy, and it forms part of the 20% body transformation plan.

So, what's so important about staying hydrated?
We can live only a few days without water - maybe a week. If you don't drink water, you die. It's as important as that!

When it comes to body transformation, water is important for the proper circulation of nutrients in your body. Water serves as the body's transportation system, and when we are dehydrated, things just can't get around as well, and it slows down your metabolism, amongst other things.

Why Is Hydration Important for Weight Loss?
Water acts as an appetite suppressant. By drinking lots of water, you will begin to consume fewer calories because water flushes out your system, cleansing your body, and reduces your hunger. Not getting in enough water can be one of the reasons why you are not breaking down body fat.

Water helps muscles, connective tissues, and joints to move correctly. It also helps the lungs, heart, and other organs to work effectively as they ramp up activity during exercise. Being hydrated while you exercise reduces the risk of muscle cramps and fatigue.

Water helps to remove waste from the body, so when the body is dehydrated, it cannot remove waste as it should. Water also helps the kidneys to filter toxins and waste while the organ retains essential nutrients and electrolytes.

Water is necessary to burn fat; without water, the body cannot properly metabolise stored fat or carbohydrates. Drinking enough water will help your body to burn off fat from food and drink, as well as stored fat.

How Does Hydration Build Muscle?

If you want to build muscle, then you must keep your body well hydrated. Water balance is a very important aspect of building muscle and the maintenance of good health.

Although water does not provide energy in the same way carbohydrates and fats do, it plays a very important role in energy transformation. When you drink the appropriate amount of water, your muscles become energised, allowing you to be more awake, alert, and train at a higher level.

You must drink water for health and building muscle. Water provides electrolytes to your muscles and without these, your muscle control and strength are weaker.

How Much Water Should I Drink Every Day?

There isn't a set amount of water that everybody should drink in a given period because the amount that it takes to hydrate one person is different from the amount that it would take to hydrate another person.

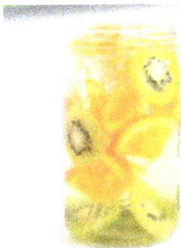

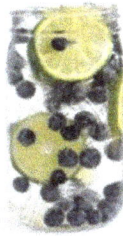

ORANGE • KIWI   BLUEBERRY • LIME   LEMON • CUCUMBER

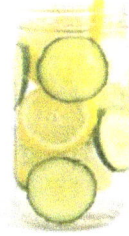

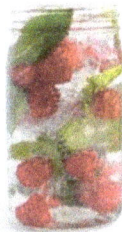

RASPBERRY • MINT   STRAWBERRY • BASIL   THE EVERYTHING

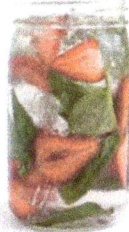

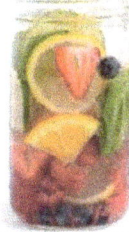

Factors that determine how much water we should drink include body composition, activity level, and water loss through sweating and breathing.

Use your body scanning scale to track if you are drinking enough water. The amount of water in your body depends on various factors, including age, gender, physical activity, and even where you live.

Drink water at regular intervals regardless of whether you feel thirsty or not. Keeping well hydrated is a must if you want to build muscle. So, to make sure that you are getting enough fluids throughout the day, drink 8 to 12 glasses of water. Drink at least two glasses of water when you wake up. Your body is in a dehydrated state after a long sleep and needs water.

Now that you know some codes for nutrition and hydration to transform your body, do you have any new plans for your body transformation goals? Is there anything you want to change about your goals?

Even though you may have tried many times to create new eating and drinking habits and not succeeded, are you ready to give it another try with these codes?

"Our Greatest Weakness Lies In Giving Up. The Most Certain Way To Succeed Is Always To Try One More Time." Thomas Edison.

I know you have the ability to transform your body! I believe in you, and I know you believe in yourself.

In the next chapter, I'm going to show you how to code your body for movement.

Congratulations on reaching this stage of your body transformation journey...... we still have 4 more codes to go!

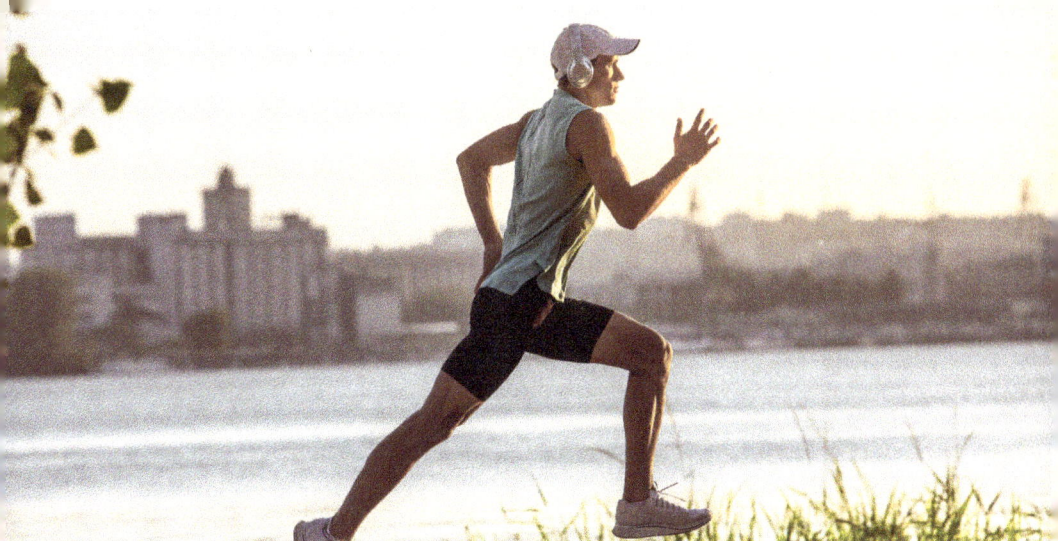

CHAPTER 3
THE MOVEMENT CODE

Our bodies are products of what we repeatedly do, good or bad.
Anonymous

Are you still with me?

How do you feel about nutrition and body transformation now that you have read the first set of coding you have to do for body transformation? Have you learned something new? Were you on the right track with what you have been doing? Or do you need to start a new set of coding because what you were doing was not giving you the results you wanted to see? Remember, nutrition and hydration are a very important part of transforming your body. If you combine these codes with movement, you have a stronger chance of transforming your body.

In this chapter, I'm going to tell you about movement. I'm going to give you specific exercises for body transformation, stretches, and some isometric exercises. These are only some forms of movement; there are many more you could use.

What is Movement?

To transform your body- you have to move, and movement is 20% of the body transformation codes.

Functional movements are movements we do as a normal part of our day, like walking and doing activities around the house like gardening and cleaning.

Movement also includes exercising at the gym or participating in sporting events like running, walking, cycling, and swimming. They also include adventure sport like river rafting, paragliding, and abseiling.

If you are trying to build or maintain muscle mass, movement is the best way because, if you don't move and use your muscles, they lose strength and size.

If your goal is to lose weight, then the movement will help you to burn calories and excess body fat.

Is going to the gym the only way to move?
No.

Walking is one of the best ways of movement you can do. Take a walk around the block, walk to the shops, park a few meters away from the entrance from where you are going so you can get to walk more often.

Do activities around your house like working in your garden, cleaning, and washing your car; all these help you move and build your fitness and lose weight. Be creative and find different activities that will get you to move.

What Happens When We Don't Move Enough?

Life has become structured in a way that makes it very easy to avoid movement. We drive to work or take some form of transport; then we sit at our desks behind computers or in meetings for most of the day. Then we come home and sit down to relax, watch TV. This is not what our bodies are built for.

Spending most of the day seated, either at work or at home, means that we face the risk of having a low metabolism rate, increased chances of back pain, becoming obese, developing posture problems and muscle degeneration, to name just a few problems associated with the lack of movement.

Why don't I see results, even when I exercise regularly?

In my experience as a Personal Trainer, having worked in various gyms and fitness centres, I have found that most people cancel their gym membership because even though they are at the gym training hard every day of the week, they don't get the results they were expecting. What happens is, they get discouraged, stop going to the gym and give up.

One of the problems is that by using before and after marketing pictures of people that have transformed their bodies, most people think that going to the gym alone is a body transformation solution.

Remember, this was my experience, too, and this is what inspired me to write this book. I want to help people like you to have an understanding of the coding that you need to have a complete body transformation so that you can get the results you are looking for, feel great, and have a great quality of life.

So, is the only way to get results through a Personal Trainer?

Personal Trainers have the knowledge, skills, experience, and abilities to design safe and effective body transformation programmes for you. They help to:

They help to:

- ✓ assess your health and fitness and can support you to set realistic personal health and fitness goals.
- ✓ Motivate and educate you.
- ✓ Reduce the risk of injury because they supervise your training
- ✓ Keep you accountable,
- ✓ Keep your training regularly, especially when you don't feel like training
- ✓ Stretch and encourage you to train optimally in each session.

But you can also get results without a Personal Trainer with good self-motivation, discipline, and consistency.

As I have worked for many years on developing programmes for my clients, I'm going to give you a set of exercises that will help you get the results you want.

If you have completed the mini fitness test in the first chapter of this book and recorded your results, you have a good idea of your fitness and strength levels. No matter where you're starting from, the more you move, the sooner you will start to transform your body.

Be sure to always consult with your doctor before starting a new exercise programme.

So, are you ready to get started?

Warm-Up

Before you start any movement, you should warm-up.

By warming up, you are preparing your body for exercise. As your body temperature increases, you'll loosen your joints and increase blood flow to your muscles. That means you will put less stress on joints and tendons.

A good warm-up will lubricate your joints and prepare your body to move with ease.

How do I warm up?

Some easy ways to warm up is to walk around the block for 15 minutes or walk up and down the stairs 10 to 30 times or walk around your house a few times.

Once you have warmed up enough, you are ready to start.

<u>Chair Squat</u>

Sit on a steady chair and stand up. Breathe out as you stand and breathe in as you sit. Repeat the movement 10 times.

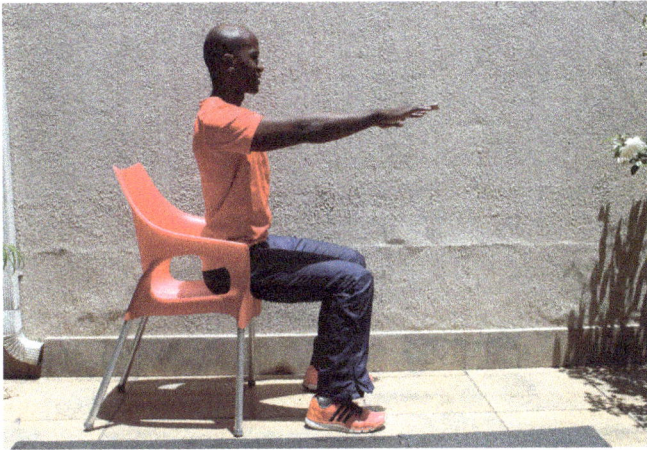

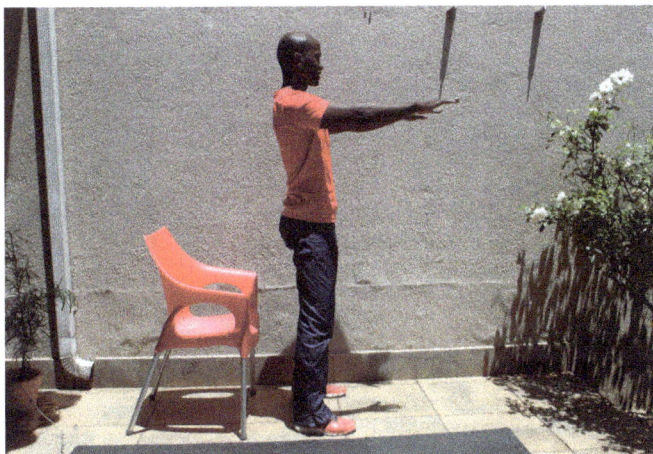

Wall Press

- Bend your elbows and lean on the wall keeping a straight back and straighten the elbows back to the starting position.
- Breathe in as you bend your elbows and breathe out as you straighten them.
- Repeat the movement 10 times.

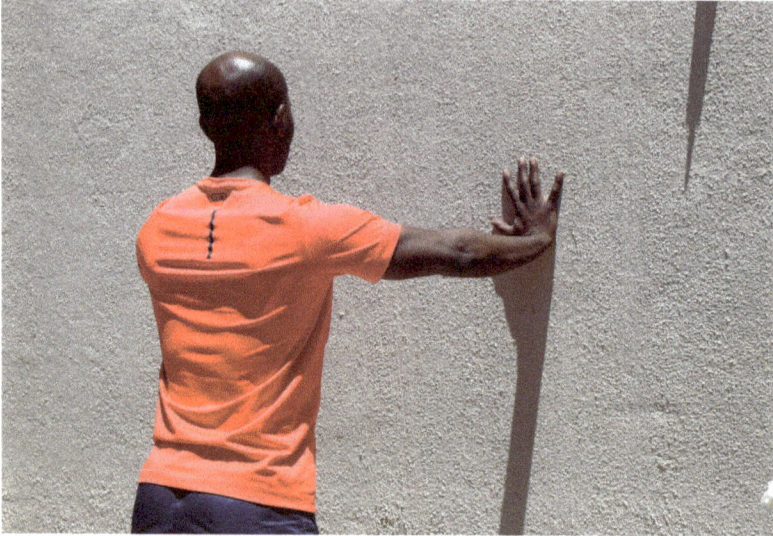

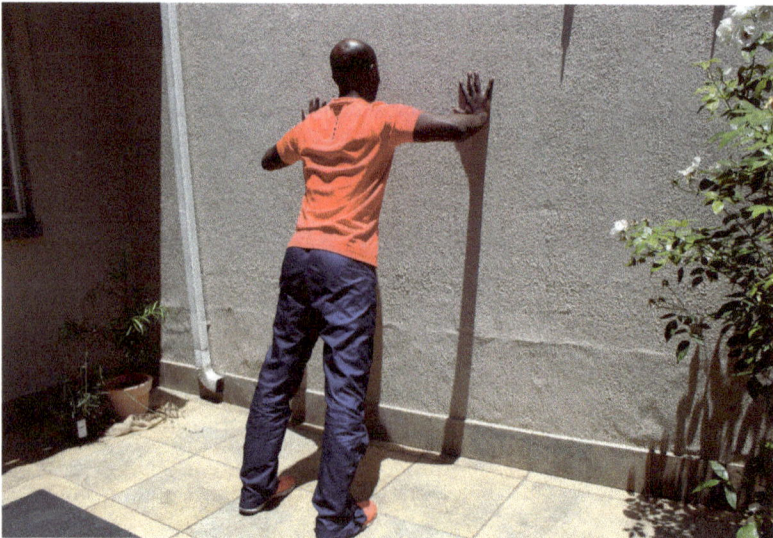

Standing Calf Raises

- Lift your heels off the floor. Hold the position for 1 second and slowly lower your heels back down.
- Breathe in as you lift your heels and breathe out as you lower them back to the floor.
- Repeat the movement ten times.

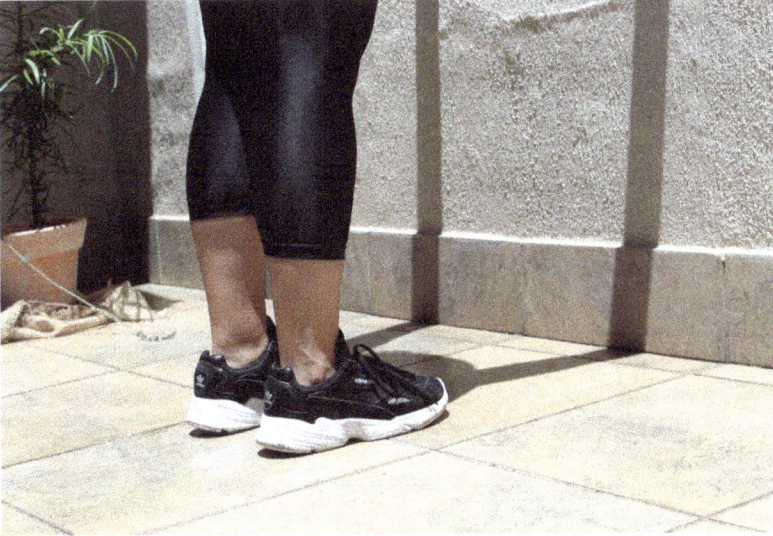

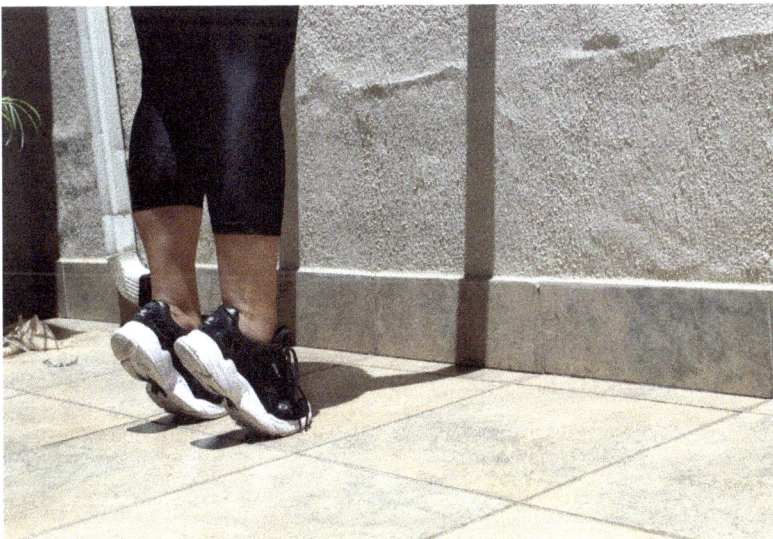

Sit-Ups

- Lie down with knees up off the floor and slowly lift the head and shoulders off the floor and hold for 1 second.
- Rollback to the starting position.
- Breathe out as you lift your head and shoulders, and breathe in as you roll back to the starting position.
- Repeat the movement 10 times.

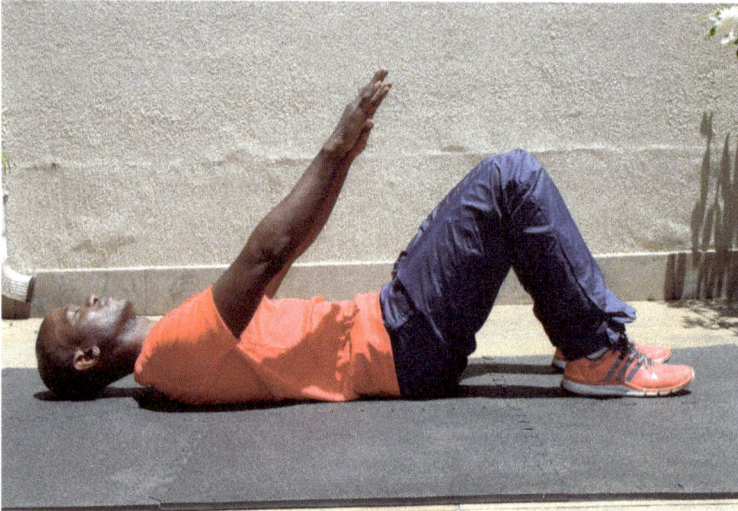

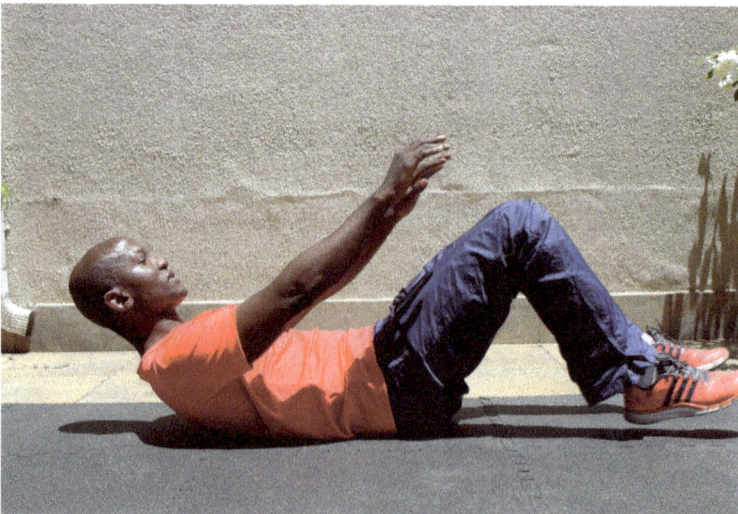

Plank

- Leaning on your elbows facing the floor, tighten your stomach muscles, and lift your hips off the ground and hold this position for 30 seconds.
- Breathe normally as you hold the position.

Leg Stretches

- Lying on your side, grip the top leg with your top arm, and stretch it backwards, holding for 20 seconds.
- Roll on to your other side and change legs.

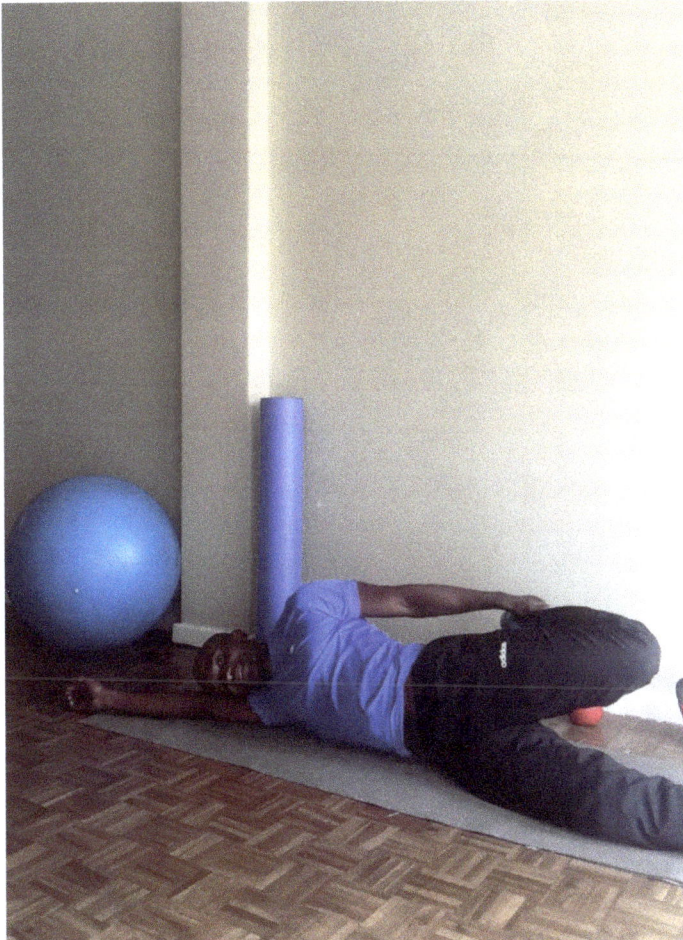

Arm Stretches

- Lift your left arm, grip it with your right, and stretch it down your back.
- Hold the stretch for 20 seconds and then change arms.

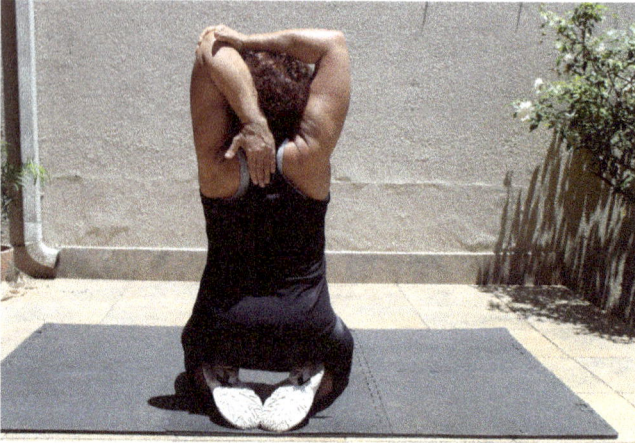

Standing Leg Stretches

- Distance your feet slightly and lean forward to touch your toes, keeping your back straight. Bend your knees slightly.
- Breathe out as you go down and hold for 20 seconds.
- Come up and repeat.

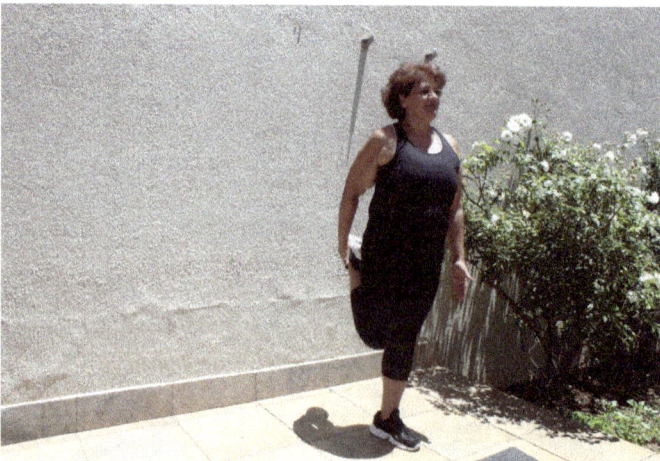

WALL AND CHAIR STRETCHES

Door Stretch
Purpose: Improve chest flexibility

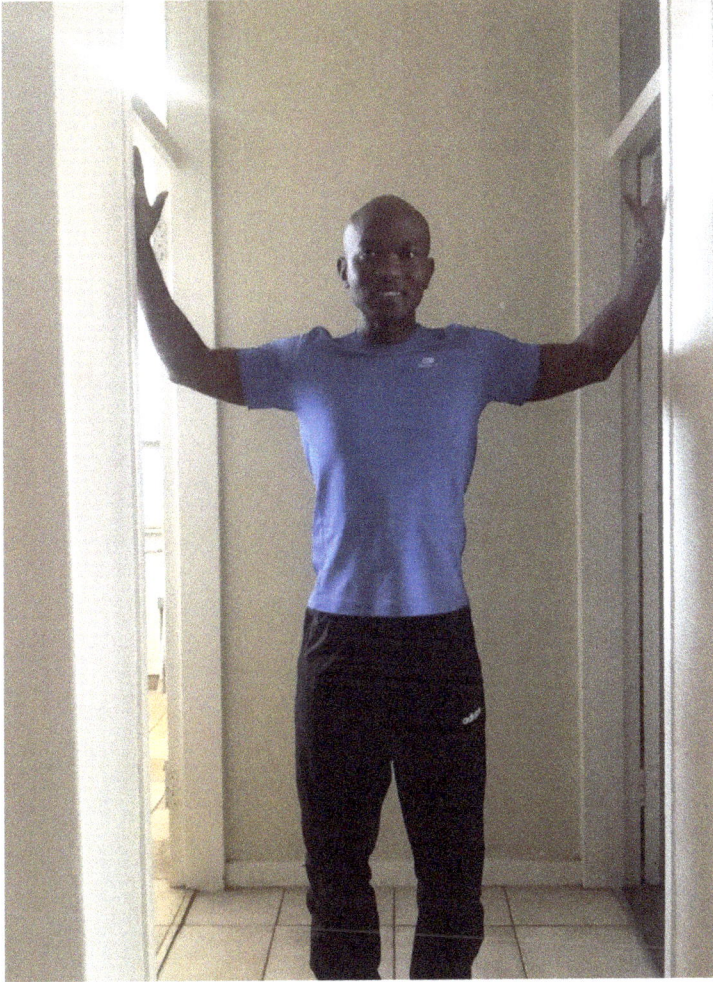

How to perform: Stand up straight and relax the shoulders.

Tip: Lean as far forward as you can and hold the stretch for 30 seconds and breathe.

Chair Stretch

Purpose: Improve leg muscle flexibility

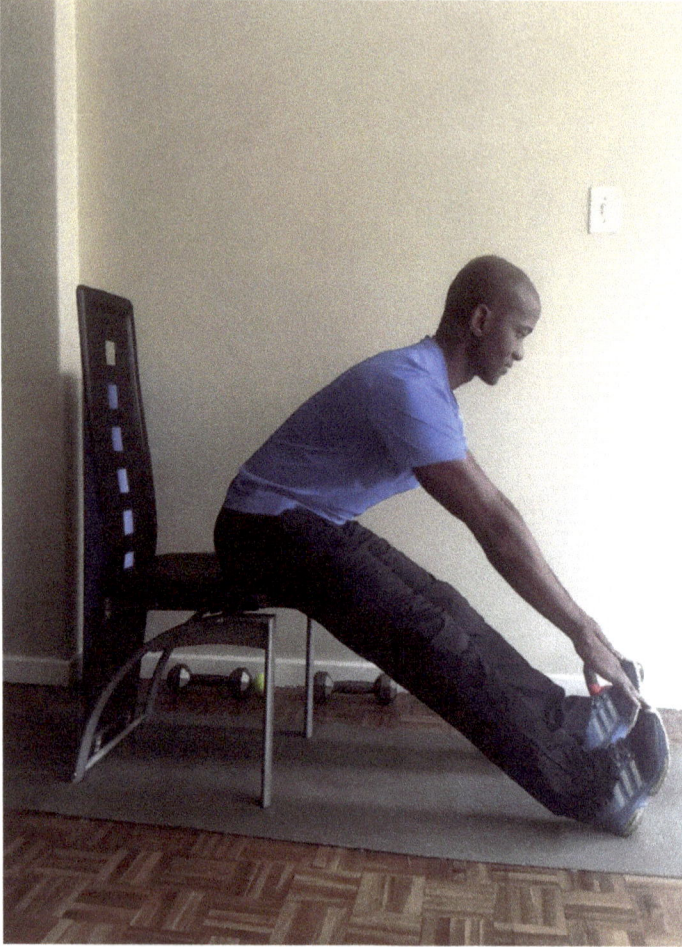

How to perform: Keep your back straight and lean forward to touch your toes.

Tip: If you cannot reach the toes, place your hands on your knees or shins.

Hold the stretch for 30 seconds and breathe.

Chair Back Stretch
Purpose: Improve back muscle flexibility

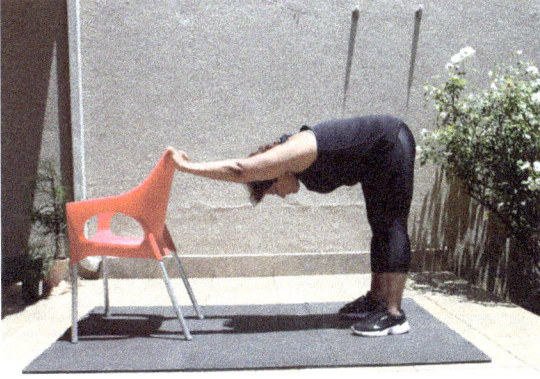

How to Perform: Hold on to a chair with straight arms, back, and straight knees.

Tip: Hold the stretch for 30 seconds and breathe.

Chair Supine Stretch
Purpose: Improve stomach and chest flexibility

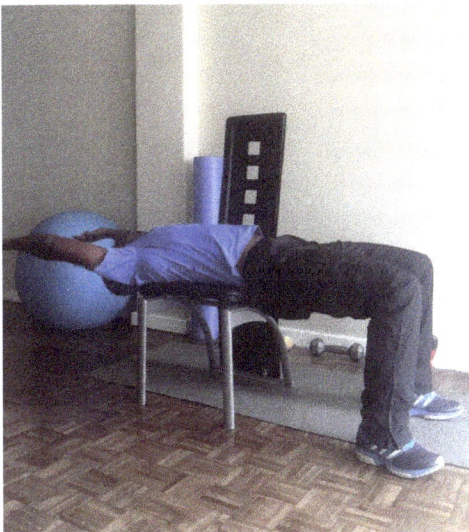

How to perform: Your feet should be shoulder-width apart. Stretch your arms as far back as you can.

Tip: Hold the stretch for 10 seconds and breathe. Get up slowly.

Chair Kneeling Stretch
Purpose: Stretch back and arm muscles

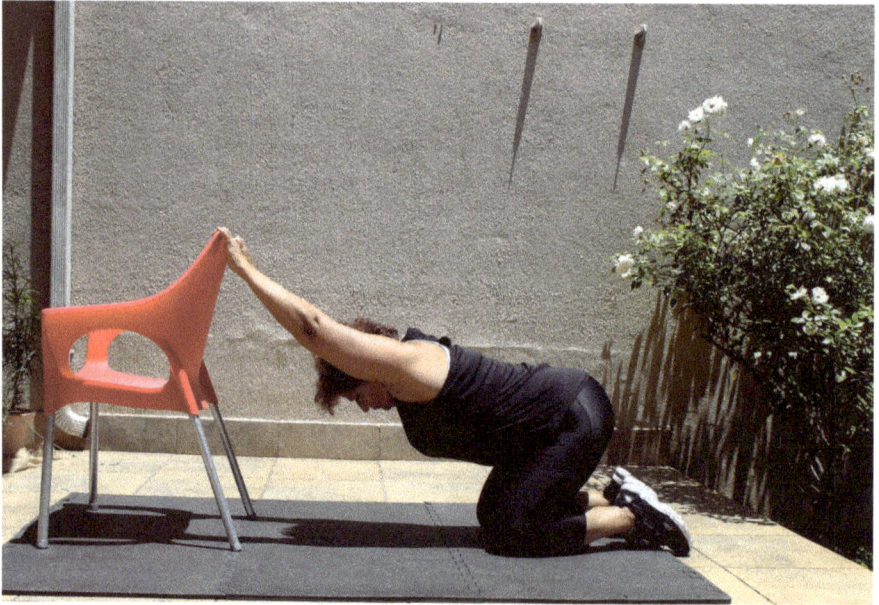

How to perform: Go on your knees and hold on to a chair.

Tip: Push your chest down as low as it is comfortable. Hold the position for 30 seconds and breathe.

Wall Arm Stretch

Purpose: Stretch arm muscles

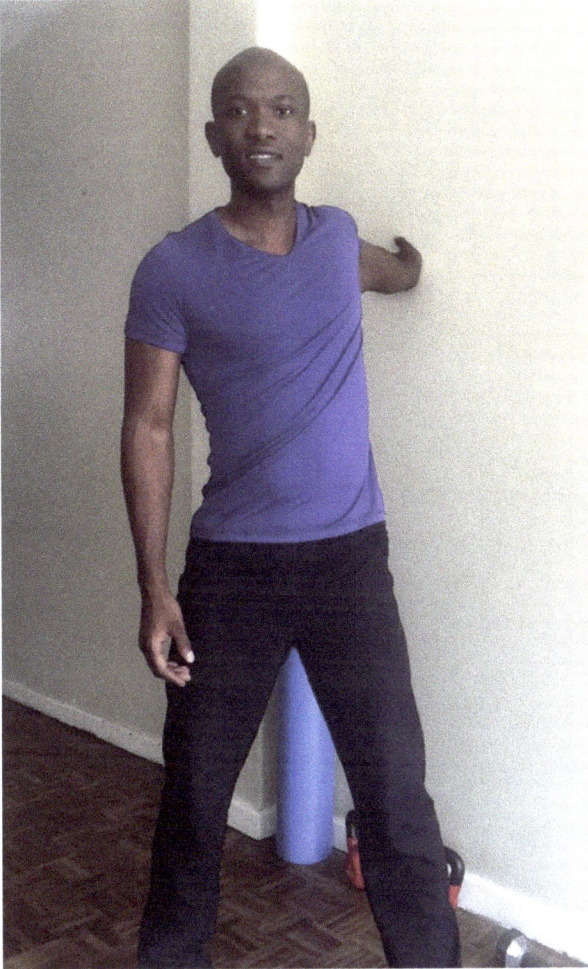

How to perform: Hold on to the wall with a straight arm and turn away from the wall as far as it is comfortable.

Tip: Hold the stretch for 30 seconds and breathe. Change arms.

Chair Chest and Arm Stretch

Purpose: Stretch arms and chest

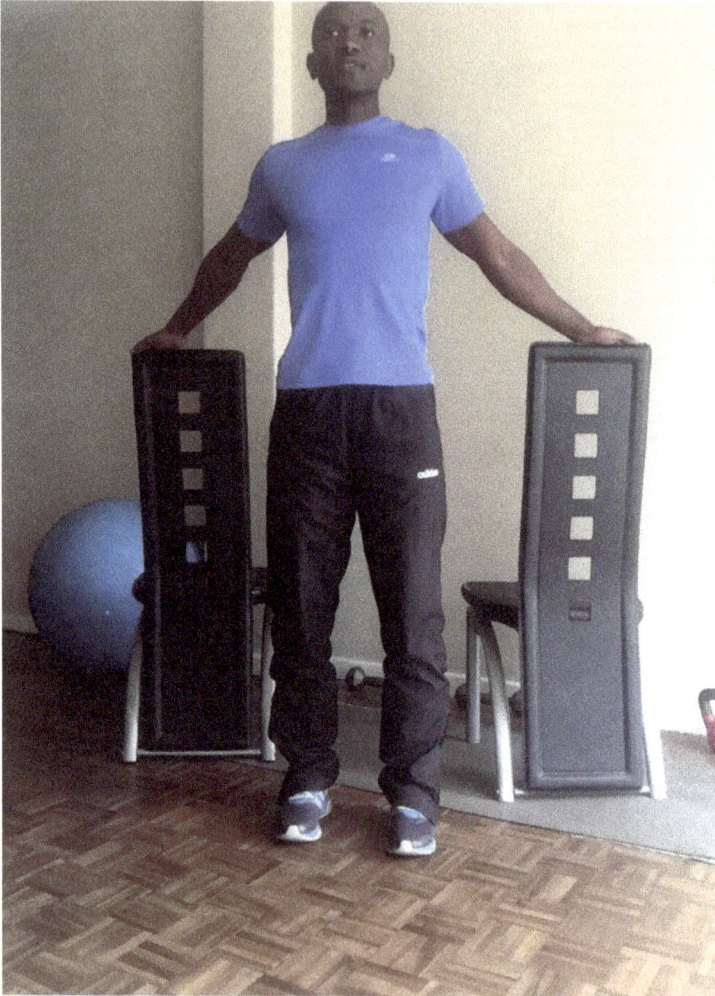

How to perform: Hold on to 2 chairs and walk forward as far as it is comfortable for you.

Tip: Hold the position for 30 seconds and breathe.

Chairs Kneeling Chest and Arm Stretch

Purpose: Is to stretch the front muscle of the body.

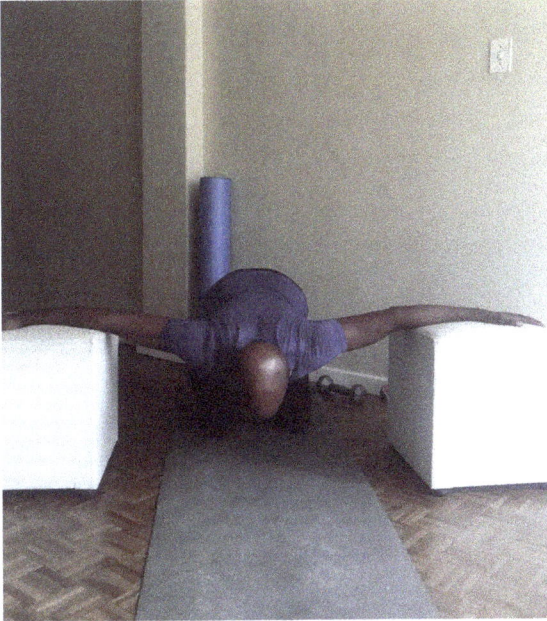

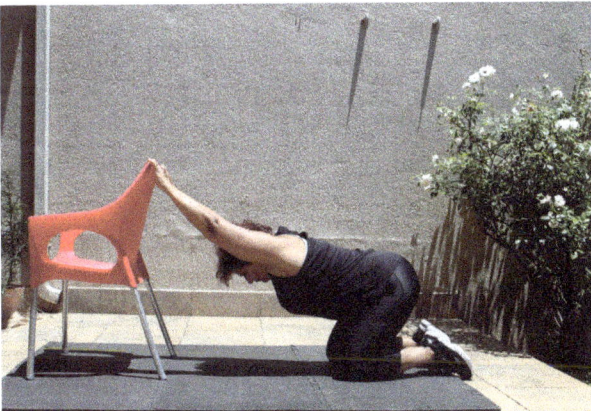

How to perform: Kneel between two chairs, and spread your arms apart, push your chest as low as it is comfortable for you.

Tip: Hold the position for 20 seconds and breathe.

Stretching Tips

- Use a stable and robust chair.
- Take short breaks between stretches.
- Drink water to stay hydrated while stretching.
- If it is too uncomfortable, hold the stretches for shorter periods.
- Do not continue with a stretch if you feel pain.
- You may progress to doing each stretch 2 to 3 times once you are fit and flexible enough.
- Stretch after exercising, taking a bath or a shower if possible because your muscle will be warm.

Isometric Abdominal Work Out

Isometric exercises are contractions of a particular muscle or group of muscles. Because isometric exercises are done in one position without movement, they'll improve your strength in only one particular area of the body. You'll have to do various isometric exercises to improve your overall muscle strength. I am going only to use an abdominal workout because this is an area that many people struggle to lose weight in or build muscle.

Exercise 1

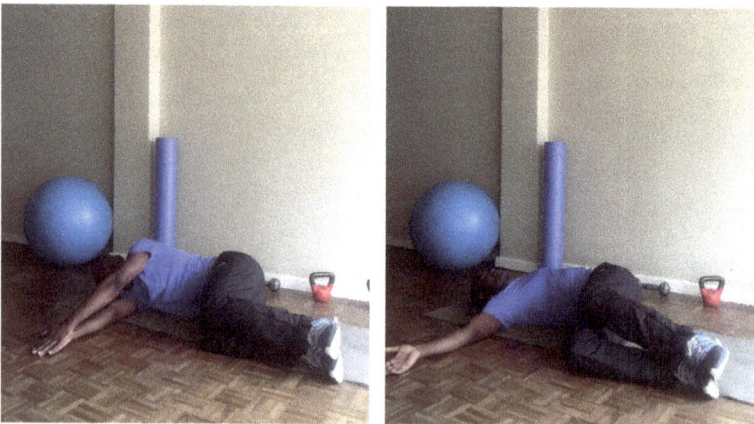

✓ Lie down on your side with your feet, knees, and hands-on top of the other.

✓ Rest your head comfortably on a pillow. As your exhale, lift your top arm and turn your head to look up. Keep the bottom arm on the floor.

✓ Both arms must be flat on the floor, and the back of your head should rest comfortably on the pillow.

✓ Return to the starting position and repeat the movement 10 times.

Change to the other side and repeat the exercise.

Exercise 2

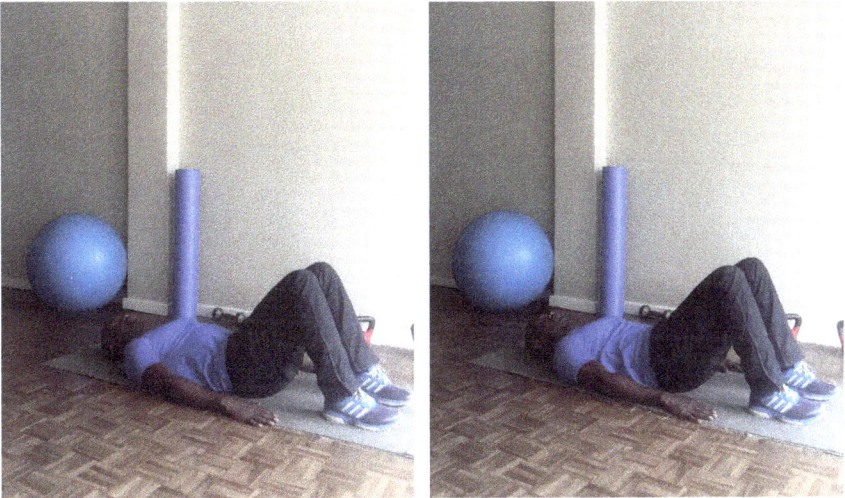

✓ Lie down flat on your back, and your knees bent at 30 degrees.

✓ Make sure your feet are flat on the mat and your legs hip-distance apart. Lay your arms flat next to your body with your palms facing down.

✓ Contract your abdominal muscles and tilt your pelvis. Make sure your lower back stays on the floor, and your buttocks are off the floor. Hold for 2 seconds.

✓ Relax your abdominal muscles and lower your buttocks back to the floor. Relax for 1 second and repeat the movement 10 times.

Exercise 3

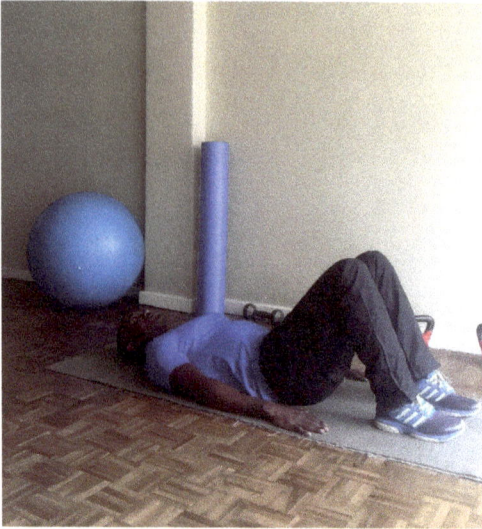

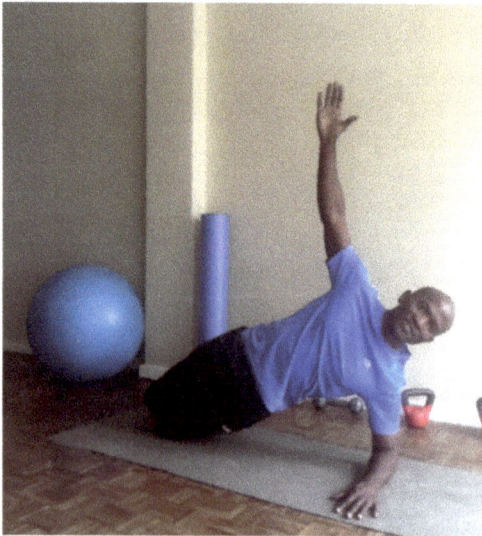

✓ Lie down comfortably on your back with your legs hip-distance apart.
✓ Lift your shoulders and your head off the mat with your hands above your thighs or knees.
✓ Hold for one minute or longer.

Exercise 4

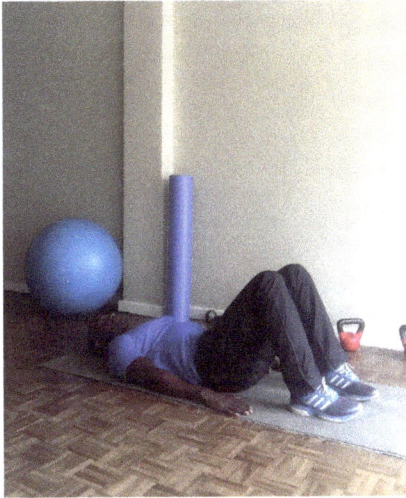

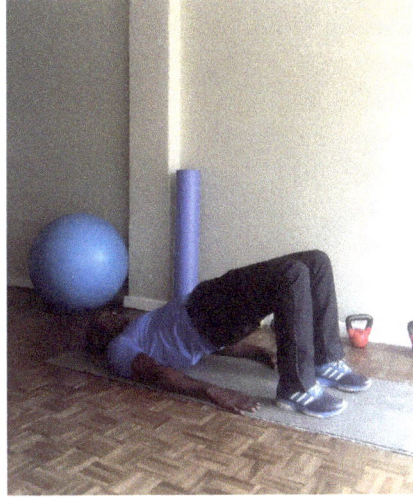

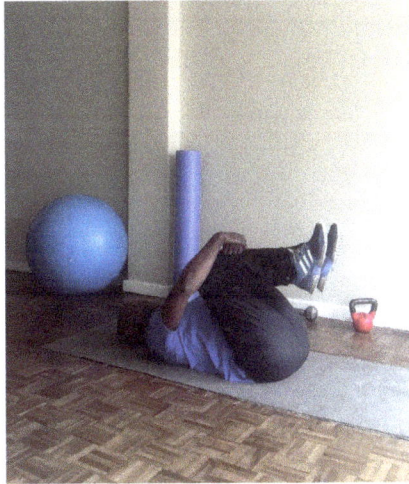

✓ Lie down on your back flat with your legs hip-distance apart and your arms flat next to your body with palms facing down.
✓ Lift your buttocks and back off the mat as high as is comfortable for your lower back. Hold for 2 minutes or as long as you can.
✓ Hug your legs and rock gently from side to side. You may keep your head down or lift it up—rock 20 times.

Exercise 5

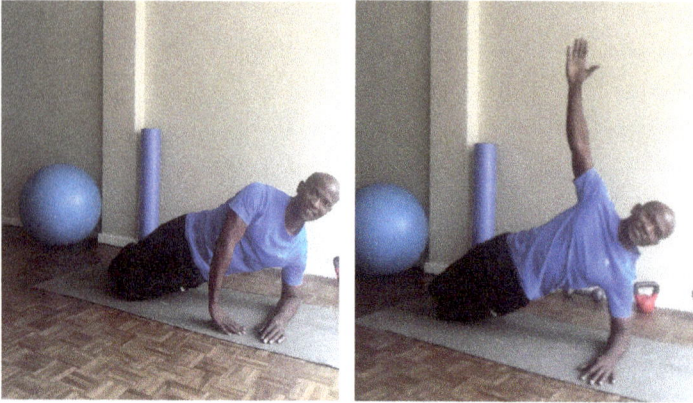

✓ On your side, make sure that your elbow is directly under your shoulder. Keep your hips, knees, and feet stacked on top of each other. Lift your hip off the mat. Change sides and repeat in the same pose.
✓ Hold for 60 seconds or longer.
✓ Turn to the other side.
✓ Hold for 60 seconds or longer.

Exercise 6

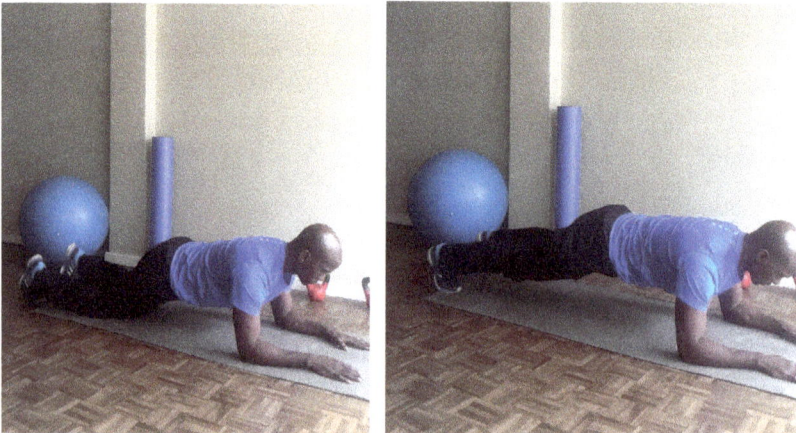

✓ Lie down on your stomach with your legs hip-distance apart; feet pointed back, elbows directly underneath the shoulders.

✓ Contract your abdominal muscles and lift your hips off the mat.
✓ Hold for 60 seconds and longer.
✓ Position your legs hip-distance apart with your feet pointed back and palms and forehead on the mat.
✓ Lift your knees and thighs as high as is comfortable for your lower back. Tighten your buttocks.
✓ Hold for 10-20 seconds.

Exercise 7

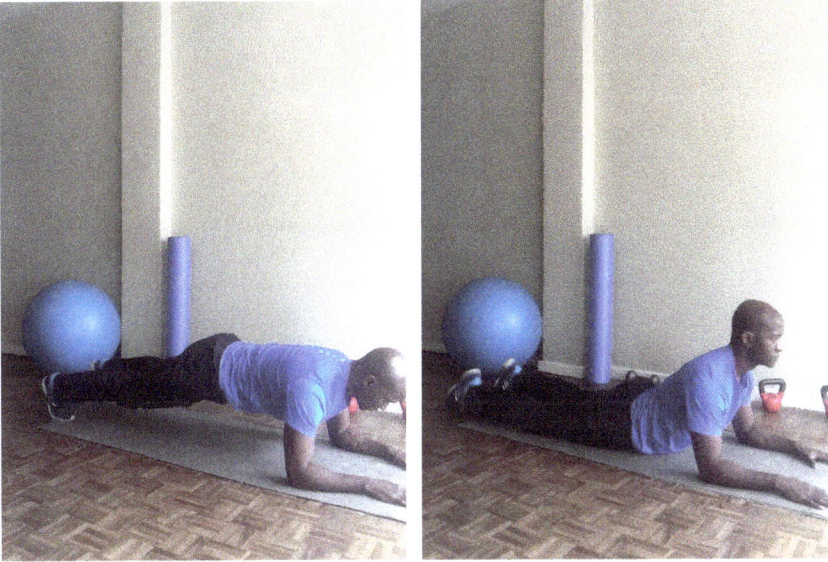

✓ Legs must be placed hip-distance apart with your elbows directly underneath your shoulders.
✓ As you exhale, tighten your abdominals, and lift your hips and knees off the mat.
✓ Hold for 60 seconds and longer.
✓ Slowly lower your knees and hips back down. Keep your elbows directly under your shoulders.
✓ Put your head up and face forward and hold this position for 20-30 seconds.

Exercise 8

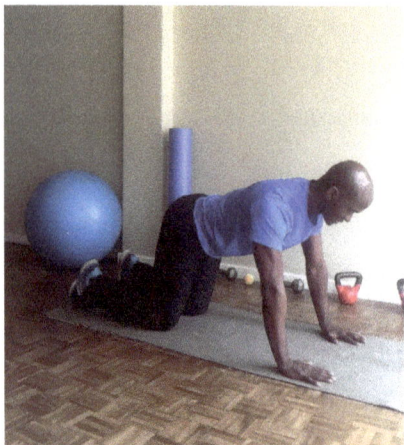

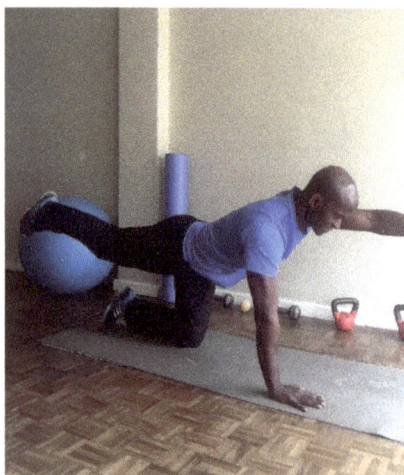

- ✓ Rest yourself on all fours with your wrists directly under your shoulders and knees directly under your hips.
- ✓ Stretch your left arm forward and your right leg back. Look down and contract your abdominal muscles.
- ✓ Hold for 60 seconds or longer.
- ✓ Stretch your right arm forward and your left leg back. Look down and contract your abdominal muscles.
- ✓ Hold for 60 seconds or longer.

Exercise 9

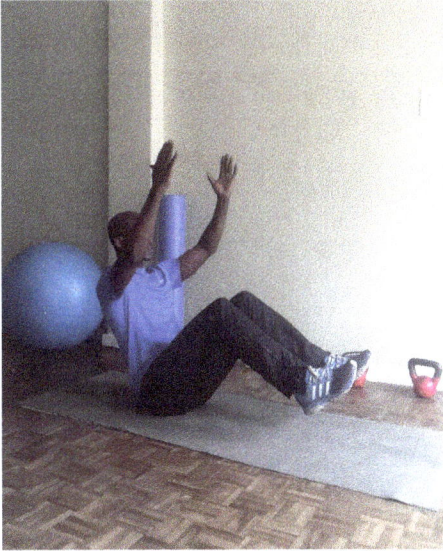

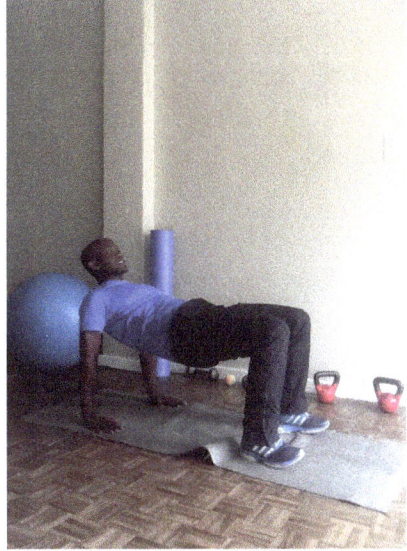

✓ From a seated position and legs hip-distance apart, lift your arms forward. The feet should be flat on the mat.
✓ Contract the abdominal muscles and relax the shoulders.
✓ Hold for as long as it is comfortable.
✓ Place your palms on the floor with your fingers pointing towards your feet. Keep your legs hip-distance apart. Lift your buttocks off the floor. Knees should be in line with your hips.
✓ Hold for 60 seconds.

So now you have a series of exercises that will help you to reach your goals. I have only given you a few exercises in this book to get you started.

For more exercises, follow me on my YouTube channel, Facebook page, and TikTok, where I demonstrate and give you information about many other body transformation exercises.

https://www.youtube.com/channel/UCy2z6Te4Y8fhqiPujHbiqGw
https://www.facebook.com/SizwePersonalTraining/videos/581679482281403/

You have now begun to code your body and mind in 2 areas – nutrition and hydration, and movement. These two coding practices should start to energise you and get you to start feeling motivated to keep going.

Remember, you can start moving no matter how you feel. Start with doing a little bit every day so that it becomes a habit; everything has to start somewhere. By participating in some movement every day, you will start to grow your confidence and fitness. It will become easier as you become more active. When you get to this stage, you are on your way to transforming your body

 If you are already fit, you should begin to see some changes in your strength, flexibility, fitness levels, and weight loss.

So now, we have gone through 40% of the 100% body transformation coding. Well done for getting to this point!

What's important is that you are working on your goals, and you can see progress. Go back to your goals and reread them. Read them every morning so that they are top of mind for you.

In the next chapter, we are going to focus on the codes for managing stress.

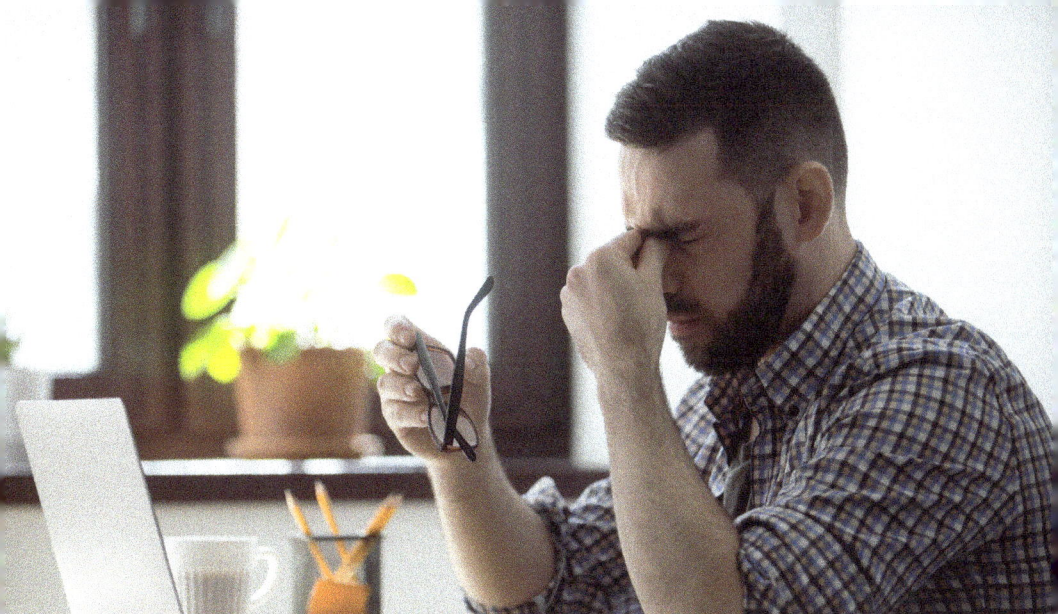

CHAPTER 4
CODING FOR STRESS MANAGEMENT

"Tension is who you think you should be. Relaxation is who you are."
Chinese Proverb

In my years of practising as a Personal Trainer, I have found that clients with demanding jobs and those who own businesses battle to transform their bodies because of stress. Some clients don't get enough sleep because of overthinking about work challenges, and they end up not having enough energy to exercise. Others turn to comfort food when they start feeling stress. As a result, they gain weight. These are some of the challenges that have prevented my clients from transforming their bodies.

I have found that to be successful in any body transformation plan; you have to learn to manage your stress.

Stress brings on the production of stress hormones, which can lead to changes in appetite and metabolization, which can cause weight loss or weight gain. But fortunately, there are many self-help techniques to decrease stress.

In this chapter, I'm going to show you the 20 % stress management code important for transforming your body. I will start by looking at what stress is and some codes for managing it through relaxation, prayer, meditation, and hobbies.

As a yoga teacher, I will go into detail about yoga Nidra as a stress management technique.

So, how do I know that I am really stressed?

Trying to explain what stress is, isn't easy. It's like trying to describe happiness. Everyone knows what it is and can feel it, but it is difficult to explain. But let's say stress is a feeling of being under too much emotional or physical pressure. Pressure turns into stress when you feel unable to cope.

If you see an event or situation as only mildly challenging, you probably feel only a little stress; however, if you find yourself in a situation or event as threatening or overwhelming, you probably feel a lot of stress. For example, having to wait for a bus when you dont have all the time in the world can trigger a little bit of stress. But waiting for a bus when you're late for an important meeting will trigger much more stress.

How do I know I am managing my stress?

You know you are managing your stress when you have a balanced life, with time for work, relationships, relaxation, and fun. You will also have the resilience to hold up under pressure and meet challenges head-on. Not all stress is bad. But long-term stress can lead to health problems.

How does stress affect Body Transformation?

1. Stress may cause you to over or under eat

Often when we are stressed, we use food to help us deal with the situation, and we do 'emotional eating.' When you're struggling to cope, we often find ourselves going over to the fridge to look for something that will satisfy our need for comfort from the stress.

For some people, it's the opposite when they are stressed; they don't eat at all.

2. Stress Throws Off Your Work Out Game

When you're facing big deadlines or coping with a family crisis, your work out sometimes falls off your list of priorities. Often, when we are under pressure, we tend to slack off on physical activity and spend more time sleeping, watching TV, or simply feeling paralyzed by the pressure.

3. Stress Prevents Weight Loss

When you are stressed, your body produces cortisol, which slows down your metabolism, making it difficult to lose weight.

How do I manage stress?

There are different ways and techniques for managing stress. Relaxing activities, praying, meditation, doing yoga are all ways of managing to stay on top of what triggers your stress levels.

Relaxing Activities

The relaxation response is the opposite of the stress response. It's a state of deep rest that you can start to tap into in many ways. If you practice these regularly, you create a place of calm to dip into when you need to.

- **Breath Focus**: Simply take long, slow, deep breaths (from your abdomen). As you breathe, gently start to take your mind off from distracting thoughts and sensations.

  Breath focus can be especially helpful to focus on your body positively.

- **Body Scan**: A body scan can help boost your awareness of the mind-body connection. After a few minutes of deep breathing, focus on one part of the body or group of muscles at a time, and mentally releasing any physical tension, you feel there.

- **Guided Imagery**: Visualise soothing scenes, places, or experiences in your mind to help you relax. If you find it difficult to visualize, there are many free apps online. Choose recordings that you find soothing, and that will help you to relax.

- **Start a Hobby**: Hobbies bring a sense of fun and freedom that can help to minimize the impact of stress. For example, you have a job or situation that is stressful and makes you feel overwhelmed. A hobby can provide an outlet for stress and something to look forward to after a hard day or week.

Prayer

- Silently repeating a short prayer or phrase from a prayer while practising breath focus can help you to destress. This may be especially helpful if religion or spirituality is meaningful to you.

- Spirituality connects you to the world, which in turn enables you to stop trying to control things all by yourself. When you feel part of something bigger than yourself, it's easy to understand that you aren't responsible for everything that happens in life, and you will start to feel calmer. You will also feel calmer if you speak to a Higher Being that is more powerful than you.

- Praying with others means getting support from your community and providing you with the opportunity to give support to others. Practising a religion provides social support, a consistent element of happiness, and good health and contributes to feeling relaxed.

Meditation

Meditation has been shown to have mental benefits, such as improved focus, happiness, and better self-control.

There isn't a right or wrong way to meditate. What's important is that you find a practice that meets your needs and complements your personality. Here are three forms of meditation you may want to try.

- **Mindfulness**: With mindfulness meditation, you pay attention to your thoughts as they pass through your mind. Don't judge your thoughts or become involved with them. Simply observe and take note of any patterns you may observe. You may find it helpful to focus on an object or your breath while you observe any bodily sensations, thoughts, or feelings. This type of meditation is good if you don't have a teacher to guide you because it can be practised alone quite easily.
- **Focused meditation:** Focused meditation involves concentration using any of the five senses. You could focus on something internal, like your breath, or you can bring in an external object to help focus your attention, like listening to a gong or staring at the flame of a candle. This practice may seem simple, but it can be difficult to hold your focus for longer than a few minutes at first. If your mind does wander, don't worry, come back to the practice, and refocus.
- **Movement Meditation:** Try a walking meditation, where you focus on paying attention to your breath and what's going on around you while you are walking. Or simply smile while you are walking. Even faking a half-smile can lower your heart rate and reduce your stress response almost instantly.

How long should I practice these techniques?

The longer and the more often you practice these relaxation techniques, the greater the benefits, and the more you can reduce stress.

Remember that relaxation techniques are skills. With any skill, your ability to relax improves with practice. Be patient with yourself.

Don't let your effort to practise relaxation techniques become another stressor.

If one relaxation technique doesn't work for you, try another technique.

Try to practice for at least 20 minutes a day, although even just a few minutes can help.

Yoga Nidra
A technique I teach and practice myself is called yoga Nidra. I learned yoga Nidra as part of the yoga teacher training style that I teach called Satyananda yoga, which is based on Swami Satyananda teachings.

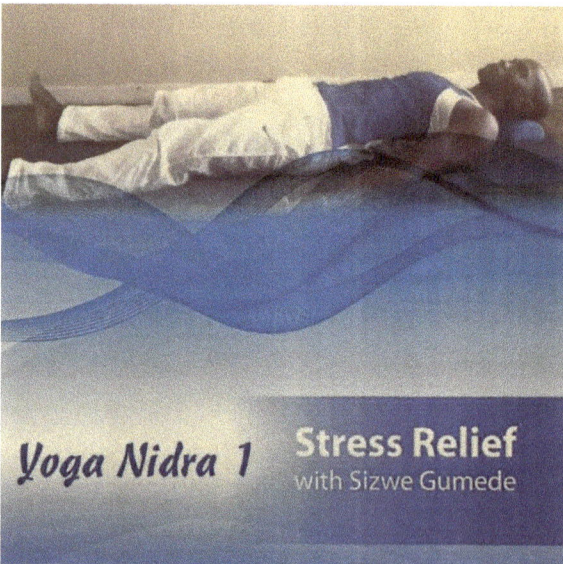

Yoga Nidra 1 — Stress Relief with Sizwe Gumede

Yoga Nidra will teach you awareness and put you in a relaxed state of mind, helping you cope with work and life stress better.

What are the benefits of practising Yoga Nidra?
Improved awareness, Decreased stress levels, A relaxed state of mind, and Improved overall health

The way to practice is to record yourself reading it and listen to the recording while you are practising. You can also get another person to read it for you while you practice.

It's not possible to read and practice at the same time.

Preparation
Let's get ready for the practice of yoga Nidra

Take off your shoes, (pause-10 sec) loosen your belt, (pause-5 sec) remove your glasses and your wristwatch (pause-10 sec)

Lie down on your back with your legs slightly apart and let your feet flop out.

Your arms must be 30 centimetres away from your body

The palms of your hands must be facing up towards the ceiling

Head in a straight line with the spine

Adjust yourself so that you are comfortable. (Pause)

During yoga Nidra, there should be no physical movement

Close your eyes and keep them closed throughout the practice

Surrender your whole body to the floor.

Relax your whole body

Say to yourself mentally; I am going to practice yoga Nidra.

I will not fall asleep during the practice of yoga Nidra

Take a deep breath in and as you breathe out, let go of all the stress and tension right into the floor (Pause)

Relaxation
Now become aware of the sounds in the distance and become aware of the most distant sound you can hear. (Pause)

Let your sense of hearing operate like a radar; move your attention from sound to sound. (Pause)

Move your mind from sound to sound; just listen; do not try to think about them, do not try to identify the source, and make your mind sensitive to hearing the sounds within the hearing range. (Pause)

Now gradually move your attention closer to sounds outside the building and then to sounds inside the building.

Now develop the awareness of this room; without opening the eyes, visualize the ceiling, floor, and your body lying on the floor. See your body lying on the floor.

Became aware of the existence of your body lying on the floor in perfect stillness

Do not fall asleep; you became aware of your body in a state of relaxation. (Pause)

Breathing

Now bring your awareness to your breath.

Observe your breath, observe your breath experience the breath in the nostrils. (Pause)

Deepen the awareness of the breath by observing the temperature of the breath. As you breathe in, feel the coolness of the breath within your nostrils, and as you breathe out, feel the warmth of the breath within your nostrils.

Complete awareness of the breath within your nostrils. As it goes in, it is cool, and as it comes out, it is warm. (Pause)

Resolve

Now it is the time to make your resolve- (a resolve is to make a commitment to doing something- for example, practising the Yoga Nidra daily)

Make a simple resolve. State your resolve clearly with feeling, faith, and awareness three times mentally. (Pause)

Rotation of Consciousness
Now we are going to rotate our consciousness through the different parts of the body. You have to move your mind from one part of the body to the next, as I name the different parts.

Repeat the name of each part mentally after me and simultaneously visualize that part in front of your closed eyes, become aware of that part, relax that part, and then move on to the next part.

The Practice
Always begin with the right hand.

Right side
Become aware of your right hand- right thumb, second finger, third finger, fourth finger, fifth finger, the palm of your hand, back of your hand, the right wrist, the lower arm, the elbow, the upper arm, the right shoulder, the armpit, the right rib cage, the right hip, the right thigh, the kneecap, the right calf muscles, the shin, the right ankle, the right heel, the right big toe, second toe, third toe, fourth toe, fifth toe, 5 toes together, the whole right foot. The whole right side, the whole right side, the whole right side. Relax the whole right side of the body

Left Side
Now bring the awareness to the left side of the body

Become aware of your left hand, the left thumb, second finger, third finger, fourth finger, fifth finger, the palm of the hand, the back of the hand, the left wrist, the lower arm, the elbow, the upper arm, the left shoulder, the left armpit, the left rib cage, the left hip, the left thigh, the left knee cap, the calf muscle, the shin, the left ankle, the left heel, the left big toe, the second toe, the third toe, the fourth toe, the fifth toe, 5 toes together the whole left foot: the whole left side, the whole left side, the whole left side. Relax the whole left side of the body.

Back
Now bring the awareness to the back of the body

The right buttock, the left buttock, right shoulder blade, the left shoulder blade, the spine, the back of the head, the top of the head, the whole back, the whole back, the whole back. Relax the whole back.

Front
Bring your awareness to the front.

Become aware of the forehead, the right eyebrow, the left eyebrow, the right eyelid, the left eyelid, the right ear, the left ear, the right cheek, the left cheek, the nose, right nostril, left nostril, the upper lip, the lower lip, teeth, tongue, the chin, the throat, the chest, upper abdomen, right abdomen, left abdomen, lower abdomen, the navel, the whole trunk, the whole trunk, the whole trunk. Relax the whole trunk.

Major Parts
The whole right arm, the whole left arm, the whole right leg, the whole left leg, the back, the head, the whole body, the whole body, the whole body. Relax the whole body completely. Became aware of the whole body completely, the whole body lying on the floor. (Pause)

Awareness of Sensation

Heaviness
Now just imagine in your mind that the body is becoming very heavy.

Awaken the idea of heaviness in the body. Gradually feel that the body is becoming heavier and heavier. The head is becoming heavy. Both arms and shoulders are heavy. The back is heavy. The buttock is heavy. The whole body is heavy. Then gradually relax part by part.

Lightness
Now feel your whole body becoming lighter and lighter. The head is light. Both arms and shoulders are light. The back is light. The buttocks are light. The whole body is light.

Heat
Now imagine you are out in the sun and you feel intense heat. Now your whole body should experience the heat of the hot tropical sun. Awaken the experience of heat as vividly as possible.

Cold
Now your body is experiencing the cold winds that blow from the mountains. The same cold one feels in the deep freezer. The experience of cold awakens the experience of cold.

Now relax your whole body. Feel your body going back to its normal temperature. Your body feels relaxed.

Visualization
Now bring your awareness to the eyebrow centre.

Now you have to visualize the objects as I name them. Visualize the object as I name them in the space in front of the closed eyes.

If I name the symbol of the rising sun, then mentally, you have to visualize the image of the rising sun in the space in front of your closed eyes- as clearly as possible and as colourful as possible.

Intensify your imagination and quickly follow the vision of the item which is being named.

The rising sun, the rising sun, the rising sun behind the mountains, the blue sky, the blue sky, white clouds, hot air balloon, the setting sun, the setting sun behind the ocean, the waves, the white waves, the beach sand, the beautiful beach sand, the moon, the full moon, the stars, a house, chimney smoke rising from the house, a car, a moving car, a river, a boat, a moving boat in the river, a garden, a garden with beautiful flowers, roses, different coloured roses, pink roses, red roses, yellow roses, smell their fragrance, the trees, the trees, a small clearing between the trees, a bench between the trees, go to the bench (Pause 5 sec),

Sit down on the bench, close your eyes, visualize yourself sitting down on the bench (Pause 5 sec), a sense of peace and harmony envelops you as you close the eyes, you are in a meditative state, feel and experience the peace and harmony. (Small Pause)

Now bring your awareness back to the space in front of your closed eyes.

Bring your awareness to the dark space in front of your closed eyes. The space in front of your forehead, watch the space, the inner space, watch the space with detachment.

Rest your mind in this warm and friendly darkness. If thoughts occur, let them come and then go, but you have to continue watching the dark space, the warm space, the friendly darkness. Continue observing the dark space with detached awareness, feeling, and experiencing relaxation.

Resolve
Now repeat your resolve 3 times. The same resolve which you made at the beginning of the practice. Repeat it mentally 3 times using the same words and the same attitude. Became aware of the resolve with feeling and with faith.

Finish
Now become aware of the breath.

Become aware of the natural breath. Experience the movement of breath in the body. Become aware of the whole body, become aware of the room, the walls, the ceiling. Become aware of the noises in the room and the noises outside the room. Externalize the mind, do not open the eyes. Become aware of the outside sounds. Gradually begin to move your body, do not rush, take your time, move your fingers and toes. Bend both your knees slowly, roll the whole body onto your right side, open your eyes slowly, and gently sit up.

The practice of yoga Nidra is complete.

Can Stress Management Really Promote Better Health And Fitness?

Stress management starts with knowing the sources of stress in your life. But this isn't as straightforward as it sounds. It's easy to identify major stressors such as moving to a new house, changing your job, going through a divorce, or losing a loved one. Pinpointing the source of your stress can be more complicated.

It's all too easy to overlook how your own thoughts, feelings, and behaviours contribute to your everyday stress levels. Sure, you may know that you're constantly worried about work deadlines, but sometimes it's because of procrastination rather than the actual job demands that causes the stress.

So how will I benefit from learning to manage stress?

Effective stress management helps you break the hold stress has on your life so that you can be happier, healthier, and more productive.

Once you get a few stress management techniques under your belt and you have done them enough times so that they become automatic, you will feel pretty fantastic when you feel totally relaxed.

Remember, the ultimate goal is to have a balanced life. This means you have time for work, relationships, relaxation, and fun—and most of all, the resilience to hold up under pressure and meet challenges head-on when they pop up.

But stress management is not one-size-fits-all. That's why it's important to experiment with different techniques and find out what works best for you.

Just like the other codes for nutrition, hydration, and movement, you have to get the right stress management coding for your body that will help YOU manage YOUR stress.

"You can't always control what happens outside, but you can always control what goes on inside."

Wayne Dyer

If you know, you have many stressors in your life, set a goal to manage your stress.

In the next chapter, I'm going to tell you how to code rest and recovery for body transformation.

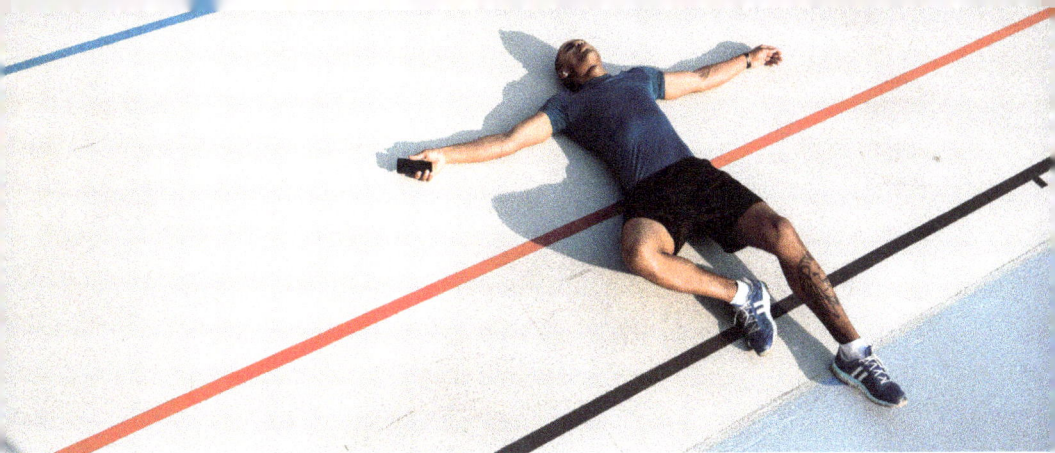

CHAPTER 5
THE REST AND RECOVERY CODE

Muscles are torn in the gym, fed in the kitchen, and built in bed.
Anonymous

I have often battled to teach clients about the rest and recovery codes, especially those who have already transformed their bodies and are working on maintenance. I guess some of them also get addicted to muscle pump like I was, or they worry about having a relapse and losing what they have developed.

Clients who do include recovery tend towards active recovery instead of taking time off to rest and recover completely and fully.

Whatever your health and fitness goals are and how much time you spend exercising and training, 20% of your plan needs to include rest and recovery.

In this chapter, we are going to talk about two aspects of rest and recovery. The first one is how to recover after training, and the second is sleep as a form of rest and recovery.

But first, let's start with an explanation of the difference between rest and recovery.

Rest and Recovery

These two words, "rest" and "recovery," mean different things for health and fitness. Both are important parts of your body transformation programme. The most important reason for including this in your programme is that during rest and recovery periods, your body has a chance to adapt to the stress associated with exercise. You have to think about both rest and recovery to keep your body safe from injury and to ensure you build your fitness free from injury.

Why are Rest And Recovery Days Important?

I'm sure that, like me, you will find that training can become addictive. Once you have caught the training bug, it can be hard to stop. However, rest and recovery days are vital if you want to achieve a high level of fitness, lose, or gain weight safely, stay injury-free, and stay motivated enough to keep working towards your health and fitness goals.

Rest and recovery are an important aspect of an exercise programme because it allows your body time to repair and strengthen itself in between workouts. It also allows you to recover, both physically and psychologically.

Your body needs time to repair and strengthen itself in the time between workouts. Continuous training can actually weaken even the strongest, fittest person. Have you noticed that your trainer sometimes gives you 'easier' days here and there in your training programme? That's because they know how important it is to have recovery days.

Physical rest is necessary so that the muscles can repair, rebuild, and strengthen. Building a rest day into your programme can help maintain a better balance between home, work, and fitness goals.

Recovery time in any exercise programme is important because this is the time that your body adapts to the stress of exercise. This is when the real effect of your training takes place. Recovery time allows your body to replenish energy stores and repair damaged tissues. Without sufficient time to repair and replenish, your body will continue to break down from exercise.

What Happens When You Don't Take Rest And Recovery Days?
Do you ever say to yourself, "I'm training my butt off, but I'm getting worse, not better!" If you find yourself in this situation, you may need more rest and recovery.

Without proper rest, your body and muscles don't have the necessary time to rebuild and rejuvenate. If we don't give our bodies rest days, the stress will start to add up.

When you don't rest enough, your energy goes down, your body suffers, and you could find yourself falling into an emotional and psychological downward spiral.

When you overuse your muscles, tendons, and ligaments, you begin to have a constant state of inflammation in your body and joints. The likelihood of getting injured is then increased.

What Is Rest?
A rest day is simply a chill-out day.

It is a time when you focus on rest, and you are not using a lot of effort or involved in the strenuous movement.

On rest days, you are taking a break from any form of training to allow your body the time to replenish its energy stores.

What Should I Do On Rest Days?

On a rest day, you may decide to sleep late in the morning or have a nap during the day, watch some movies on the couch, get a massage, read a book and go to bed nice and early, so you get a good night's sleep.

And to assist your body, here are some basic things to include on your rest day:

✓ Drink plenty of water
✓ Eat nutritious foods
✓ Do activities that relax your mind and body
✓ Sleep

Rest days should be part of your exercise plan, not something you do only when you remember or feel that you need it.

How Often Should I Have Rest Days?

There is no one answer to this question. The best thing to do is to discuss this with your personal trainer, who can offer advice that will suit your goals, ability, level of fitness, and the exercise programme you are on.

The number of rest days incorporated into your training plan will depend on the type of exercise you are doing and your ability level. As you get fitter, you will need smaller resting periods than when you just started.

Is One Day Of Rest Enough?

The type of exercise programme you do will impact the amount of rest time you need. Whether you are doing a strenuous exercise programme or participating in a sports event, you will require different rest periods.

The length of time required to rest and restore your body fully will vary from person to person. While you may not need a full 24 hours of rest, for someone else, this may be just the right amount of time.

It's worth repeating this - your personal trainer must advise you about resting to ensure that your rest periods are optimal following a workout.

What Is Recovery?
Recovery is far more than just taking a day off from exercising. Taking time for recovery means you are giving your body time to restore itself.

Taking a recovery day means that you are consciously choosing to do something that helps your body restore itself. When you take time to recover, your body and mind have time to offset the physical and psychological stresses from exercising.

Are Recovery Days Necessary?

Definitely!
Many of my clients believe that it is the physical act of exercise that makes you stronger. While this is true, I have come to realise, through my experience and reading that, the truth is that your body strengthens itself during recovery periods.

During recovery periods, your body has the chance to adapt to the strain it has gone through during a workout whilst simultaneously replenishing your energy stores and repairing body tissue.

How Many Recovery Days Do You Need?
As I said about rest days, there is no one-size-fits-all answer to this question. Your recovery period will depend on the type of exercise programme and your ability level.

Discuss incorporating recovery days into your exercise plan with your personal trainer. They will be able to offer advice suited to you to help you meet your fitness goals. Remember, too, they can observe you when you are exercising, and they also observe when you have not fully recovered from a strenuous session.

Why Is Recovery Time Important?
Building recovery time into an exercise programme is important because this is when the body adapts to the stress of exercise, and the real training effect occurs. Your muscles don't actually grow while you are working out; they grow while resting in between sessions.

Remember, exercise is essentially stress, and when you repeatedly stress your body, it becomes better adapted to respond to the type of exercise you are doing.

When you don't allow yourself adequate recovery time, you may have overtraining syndrome. Overtraining syndrome, or OTS, can compromise your immune system; make you feel exhausted, and cause chronic joint and muscle pain. This is what happened to me when I had mild shoulder pain.

Recovery is super important to your workout; it will help you to avoid all of those negative side effects, especially to avoid injuries.

If you dont allow your body enough time to adapt to the physical demands of training, it will never get a chance to 'catch up' and get stronger.

Different Forms Of Rest And Recovery

Active Recovery
Active recovery is doing low-intensity exercise after participating in a heavy workout. Unlike rest periods, active recovery involves

gentle exercises that help your body to recover. Active recovery helps to soothe sore muscles and repair any small muscle fibre tears that occurred during a vigorous workout.

• Active recovery allows your muscles to "gradually" slow down rather than rest all at once. This technique helps your body to alleviate the stress of intense exercise and steadily cool down.
• Active recovery, which is light exercise during the recovery phase, can stimulate blood flow to the muscles to help reduce muscle pain.
• Active recovery exercises may help avoid the crash or depressed mood you may feel in following a high-intensity workout, and it levels out heart rates, so there are no sudden stops and starts.

What kinds of Active Recovery activities can I do?
• Active recovery can include easy swimming or a light jog.
• Getting a massage helps to loosen up muscles, increase oxygen and blood flow into muscles, remove lactic acid build-up (which is what makes you sore), and deliver nutrients from your body to your muscle.
• Drinking plenty of water on recovery days can help flush out toxins from your body and prevent dehydration, which can create soreness in the muscle.
• Food helps to restore the body's energy supply, so eat good, healthy options on your recovery days to help your body along.

Recovery And Your Mind
Adding a mental practice to your workout routine can be a huge benefit for anyone trying to transform their bodies. Spending time practising a mindfulness meditation programme can help process a calm, clear attitude and reduce anxiety.

Become familiar with how your mind works, how your thought process works. Once you know how your mind works, you will be able to control it more and more to your benefit. (You can read more about this again in the chapter on Stress Management.)

Practising positive self-talk can also help change the conversation in your head, especially when you lose motivation and perhaps go through a period when you can't see results.

Mindful meditation and positive self-talk during your recovery days can help you to refocus on your goals and remember why you set them. On your recovery days, use the time to strengthen your will power to reach your goals.

Listen To Your Body
If you pay attention, in most cases, your body will let you know what it needs.

The most important thing you can do is listen to your body to know when to rest and recover. Suppose you are feeling tired, sore or notice that you do not see results. In that case, you may need more recovery time or a break altogether from exercising.

The problem for many of us is that we don't listen to those warnings or we dismiss them with our own self-talk ("I can't be tired, I didn't run my best yesterday" or "No one else needs two rest days after that workout; my trainer will think I'm not making an effort if I go slow today.")

Share how you feel with your Personal Trainer. Remember, trainers understand how to support you, and want you to succeed.

Is Active Recovery Better Than Rest?
It isn't really a question of which is better than the other. Both are important to ensuring your body restores energy and repairs and strengthens your muscles.

Sleep As A Form Of Recovery

What if I told you that an important part of an exercise plan involves sleeping?

Sleep is the most potent recovery tool known to science. Nothing else comes close to having a good sleep. If you're not getting enough sleep, there is nothing that will make up the difference.

If we don't sleep enough; after a while, we lose the coordination and function of our muscles and muscle movement patterns.

What Does Sleep Do?

Sleep is one of the most important ways to get your body to recover from the physical and mental demands of exercise quickly.

Sleep is the time when your body repairs the stress of exercising. Sleep allows the body to build and rebuild muscles.

On the other hand, sleep deprivation makes you more susceptible to injury.

The bottom line really is - sleep is your number one recovery priority.

So, What Happens During Sleep?

- Sleep gives you more than just rest for your brain. Sleep gives you more than just rest; it recharges your "battery," which means your nervous system and energy stores are replenished.
- Naturally, the deeper and better you sleep, the better you reload. That's important because if you don't let your central nervous system (CNS) recuperate, your fitness suffers, which means you become slower, weaker, maybe even less coordinated in your workout.

I struggle to fall asleep at night – what can I do?

Suppose you have a job where you work long hours, possibly on a laptop, checking emails, using your mobile phone, or catching up on news or social media late at night. In that case, you may find it difficult to fall asleep. The problem is that the blue light emitted from your devices will trick your brain into thinking it's still daytime. The best thing is to set aside your electronic devices at least one hour before you go to bed. This will help your melatonin levels naturally rise to where they need to be before you go to sleep.

Sleep rituals are important. Following a routine before going to bed will help you ease into sleep. Here are some rituals to try:

- Lie down, meditate, do some positive self-talk, read a book, or talk to another person. All of these things are relaxing and will also get your heart rate down.
- Your bedroom environment is an important factor: If you live in a city, make sure you don't have too much light from outside shining into your bedroom
- Make sure you are warm enough or cool enough so that you can fall asleep.

The bottom line is - create the optimal environment for sleep.
No matter where you are currently in your fitness, you should take time to rest and recover. It will benefit you in significant ways down the road towards your goals.

Consider trying different rituals from my suggestions and see what works for you. Different things work for different people, so find out what's best for your body.

So far, we have covered four codes that you need to transform your body.

Are you ready to learn about the last code? It's all about support and accountability.

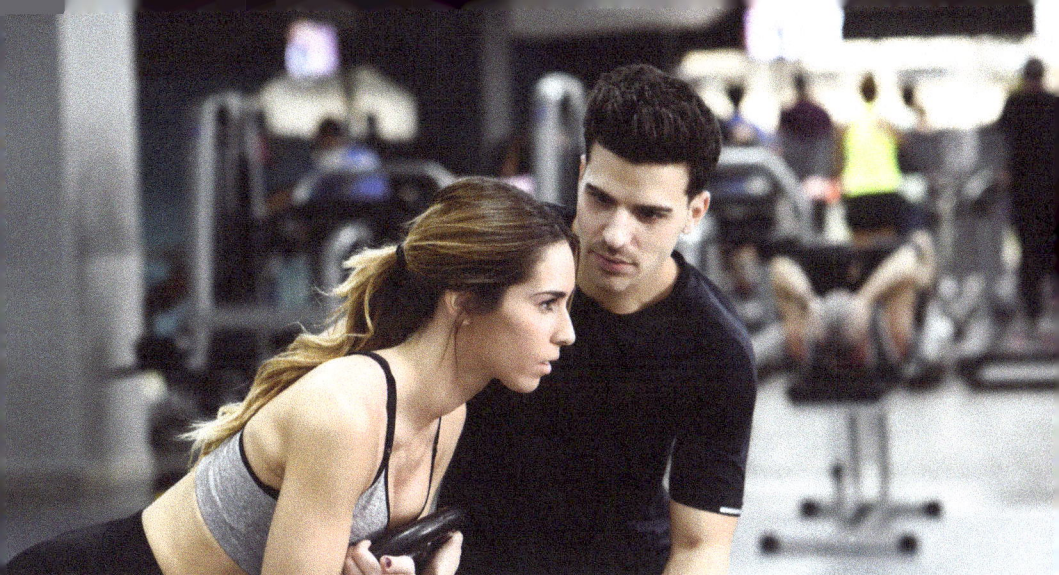

CHAPTER 6
THE POWERFUL CODES FOR SUPPORT AND ACCOUNTABILITY

If You Hang Around 9 Fit People, YOU Are Going To Be The 10th!

In this chapter, I'm going to talk about the 20 % coding that has to do with Support and Accountability. It is one of the most powerful codes for reaching your goals. With both support and accountability, you stand a much better chance of succeeding.

I discovered the support and accountability part of a body transformation when I joined a gym to work on my own body transformation. My membership meant that I could use all the machines at the gym. But I didn't know which machines to use for my specific body transformation goals. But then, with the support of a personal trainer who showed me the correct machines to use for my specific goals, I stood a better chance of succeeding.

What was important was that she kept me accountable with specific training days and coached me about the right way of eating for my body transformation goals.

You are only as Good as the Company You Keep

I also learned very fast that I had to spend less time with the people, friends, and family, who had lifestyles that were not in line with my goals. My friends wanted to drink alcohol on the weekend and stay up late. This lifestyle was not in line with my goals, and I had to make changes.

I realized that I had to start spending more time with people who were exercising and understood the idea of fuelling my body a certain way and going to bed early, even on weekends, so that I could start my training week fresh and rested on Mondays.

Every successful transformation has a *why*, and more importantly, a strong *why*. This is what allows you to focus on creating real, meaningful change. It becomes the anchor to reaching your goal and helps you get through the days when you feel like giving up.

With a strong *why* you'll know that the outcomes of what you are doing are important. This is why spending time discovering your *why* before beginning your body transformation journey will determine whether you succeed or fail.

Support

"A great way to fail is to go it alone."

We all need support at some time or another in our lives. Support means that people around you will help keep you mentally and physically strong when you're not your best.

If you have never worked out or exercised consistently for a year or 2 years or more, you will need support to get to your goals.

If you're new to exercise or have struggled to stick with it long enough to see results, you will know how important support is for your long term success.

Let me will explain how support works.

Many of my clients tell me about the "trying it on my own" method. After many, many gym memberships and lots of money spent, most have not achieved their desired results.

Some have tried to secretly make changes just "in case" they didn't succeed. The challenge is that, when you chose this approach, you have already set yourself up for massive failure.

By finding the right support, many clients have found it easier to stick with their plans.

The Power of Accountability
Accountability is having someone holding you to the "promises you've made to yourself," and it can take you a long way to helping you reach your goals.

Self-Accountability
Self-accountability is critical to any transformation journey. It forces excellence in your actions, holds you to high standards, and builds self-esteem as you tick the boxes required to achieve your goals.

By programming all the codes in this book, you are likely to have created a strong sense of personal commitment and self-accountability, and drive to reach your goals.

When you're trying to lose weight or maintain hard-fought weight loss, willpower alone often isn't enough to keep you on track. And even if you think you're maintaining your body transformation plans, it's easy for old habits to start creeping back again. Think about how many times you have lost weight, only to put it all back again. Or got fit and then lost that fitness again.

One way you can make sure you have strong self-accountability is to cultivate a growth mindset.

A growth mindset means that you stay focused on the fact that your journey is not a pass or fail. Your journey is self-exploration and getting to understand yourself better. Know what motivates you and what discourages you.

If you constantly do not do well in reaching your goals, take an honest look at the why and see how you can try a new strategy. A fixed mindset, which is too specific about the result, generally leads to you giving up because you will feel either that you "passed or failed", "won" or "lost".

What I mean about self-exploration is that beating yourself up about something you have not achieved is negative and self-defeating.

Take a minute to look at the reasons you did not produce the results you wanted, and then try a new strategy. Look at the reasons, and then let it go, dust yourself off, and get back on track.

When you take the time to think about what you have learned about yourself, you can develop new strategies to help you reach your goals.

But relying only on self-accountability will not always work, especially when things get tough. You may reach a plateau in your weight loss, or you may not be able to push through another set of pull-ups or reach the goal time for your run. Self-doubt, self-sabotage, and procrastination can set in – even when you know you have a check-in or assessment date ahead.

You could add another code to your plan to have a powerful accountability structure - peer accountability.

Peer Accountability

While your body transformation journey is your own, it's not easy doing it alone. Having a strong support system and peer-level accountability can make reaching your goals more enjoyable and create some positive pressure to achieve your goals.

Tell your family, colleagues, and friends about your health and fitness goals. Tell them what you are doing to achieve them. You may cringe when you see a friend post their health and fitness progress on social media, but what they're doing is adding another layer to their accountability systems. When you tell your family, friends, and colleagues what you're doing, why it's important to you, and what you want to achieve from it, they'll hold you accountable and support you.

Don't be afraid to ask for their support.

But it doesn't stop with self and peer support. There's one more layer that has the power to push you to your limits and achieve your goals - a personal trainer.

A Personal Trainer

A personal trainer who has a proven track record in helping people with similar goals to yours and who practices what they preach can take you a long way.

Successful people like musicians, sporting legends and personalities, even presidents of countries, have Personal Trainers. In this relationship, celebrities learn to be accountable and make sure they have the habits that will transform their bodies and reach their health and fitness goals.

A good Personal Trainer will develop the codes for your individual success and hold you accountable for taking action and making progress. He or she will show you the tools, strategies, and solutions to deal with the predictable mistakes, challenges, and obstacles everyone faces on their journey, and you'll save time and money in the process. A Personal Trainer will give you feedback on how you are doing and then encourage you to do one more. when you feel you are about to drop dead during your workout.

Remember, your challenges are not unique. Many people who try to transform their bodies go through similar failure and successes. An experienced results-producing professional Personal Trainer will support you, and provide insights into your body transformation that will help you reach your goals. It's like having an extra pair of eyes and another brain to support you.

But there is one more layer of accountability you can use.

Tribes

Tribes are groups of people who, like you, are working towards body transformation. The support they will give you is different from your peers because they are going through similar challenges to you, and they can identify with your challenges and successes. You will also find that a tribe can support you and hold you accountable at the same time.

I have started many tribes with my clients. By being part of a tribe, members support each other and hold each other accountable for goals, and what's most important, when you need motivation, your tribe is there for you.

Think about the possible support system around you, and ask yourself;
✓ Which family members, and friends will you tell your goals to?
✓ Who of your peers is likely to support you?
✓ Are there an existing tribe working towards similar goals that you can join, or if not, how can you start one?

Accountability Through Journaling
It's important during your body transformation to take the time to look inward.

I can recommend that you keep a journal for the exercises and tasks you'll work through in this book and let it evolve into your ultimate self-awareness.

By observing your thoughts and feelings through journaling, you'll be able to make sense of all the questions that your journey will bring with it. You'll gain a better understanding of yourself. And as you go in search of your "aha" moment, you'll find reasons for your previous failures and more keys to your future success.

How your journal will be is up to you. I like to spend five to twenty minutes when I wake up on one of these topics:

✓ Observing lingering and present thoughts
✓ Writing out my gratitude and appreciation
✓ Finding solutions to a problem
✓ Reflecting on my recent wins
✓ Acknowledging the progress I have made

These are some ideas to get started. Find your own style as you build momentum with journaling.

Explore the best way to identify what support you need and as a way of accounting for yourself.

Some More Ways Of Staying Accountable

Accountability is about regular checking in on where you are and making sure that you see the changes you want to make.

At the beginning of this book, in the chapter on Getting Started, you did a few assessments to set a health and fitness baseline for yourself. You also recorded information about yourself and the goals that would help you to change. Keep using this information to hold yourself accountable.

Make Friends With Your Scale

You might have a love-hate relationship with your scale — normal daily fluctuations can be maddening when all you want to see is 1 less kilogram. But it can still be a very useful tool.

Weight creeps up over time, so the best way you can keep track and make immediate corrections to your plans is to weigh yourself regularly.

Use a Tape Measure to Stay on Track

A very good way to measure success is with a cloth tape measure. By measuring your waistline, hips, bust, thighs, and calves, you can record tangible progress toward your goal with the kind of detail that a scale can't give you. Because muscle takes up less volume than fat, you'll see inches drop, even when there might not be a corresponding change on the scale. It's very empowering — and encouraging, and motivating.

Don't Keep Your Fat Pants

You may feel that you want to keep a pair of "fat pants" just in case you feel the weight starting to creep back. As for having a pair of fat pants,

I ask my clients to get rid of anything like that once they reach their goal, so they know " there's no going back."

Rather keep a different pair of pants handy — ones you know you always want to fit into. Or keep a pair of pants that you can nearly fit into to keep focused.

Create Your Own Rewards Programme

Body Transformation is a journey. So, set up little rewards along the way to keep on the right path. Maybe you have reached a dress size goal, a weight goal, or a centimetre goal; reward yourself for the mini-goal. It's another way of staying accountable. When you have reached your goal, get a massage or facial or go and see a movie. Treating and rewarding yourself will keep you in a positive frame of mind.

Support and accountability are a big part of what I do in my profession as a Personal Trainer. I create virtual groups for clients with similar body transformation goals to support each other.

I also use technology to support and keep clients accountable. I track clients' meals using apps and give tips on what they can do to support their fitness goals and achieve results fast.

Another way I support clients is through my YouTube channel and Facebook page.

https://www.youtube.com/channel/UCy2z6Te4Y8fhqiPujHbiqGw
https://www.facebook.com/SizwePersonalTraining

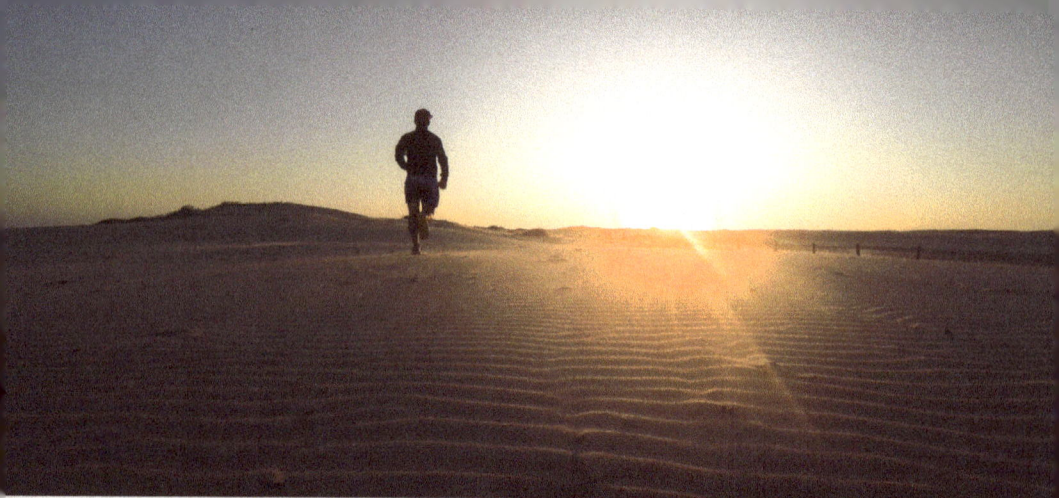

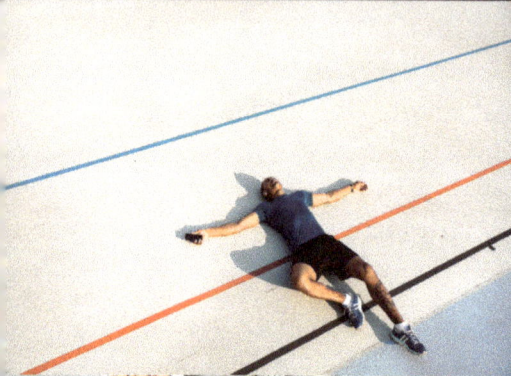

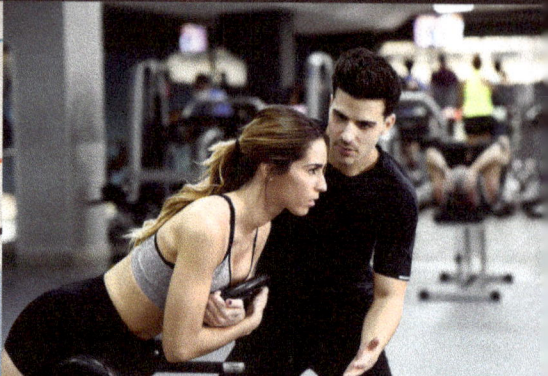

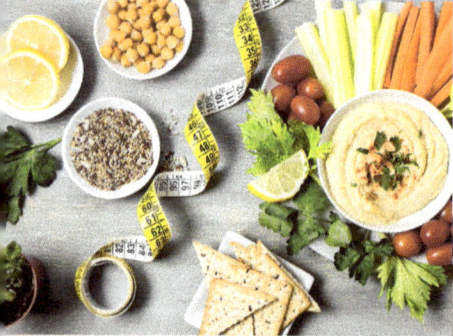

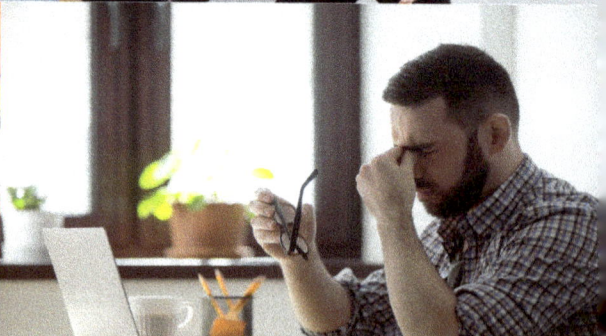

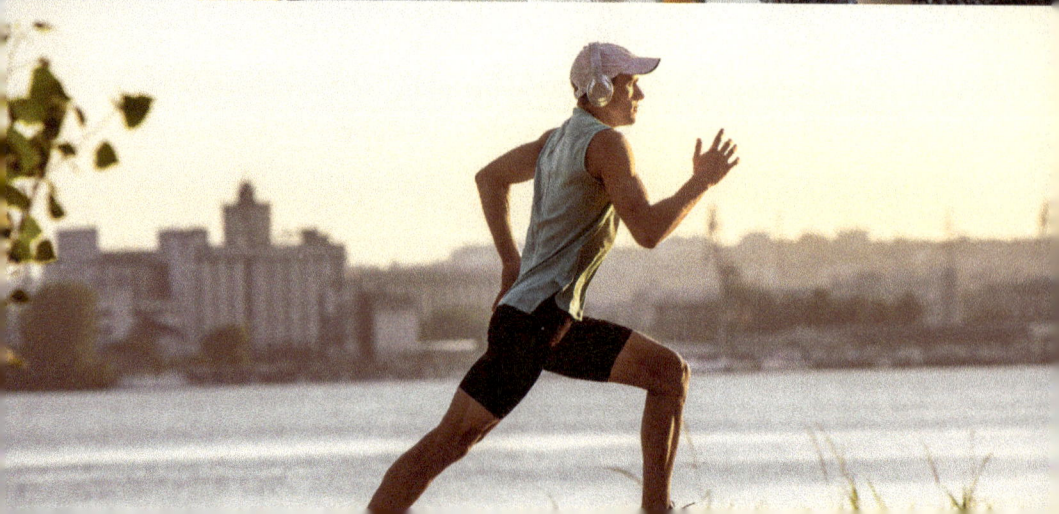

BRINGING IT ALL TOGETHER

"Motivation is what gets you started; habit is what keeps you going."
Jim Rohn

How are you feeling right now? Overwhelmed? Excited? Sceptical? Cracking these codes, as I have said, will take commitment, focus, and dedication.

Most of all, the best thing you can do to make sure you succeed is to start forming form habits that will create a body-transforming code. Good habits happen when we set ourselves up for success.

The best way to form a new habit is to link it to one of your existing habits.

Look for patterns in your day and think about how you can use existing habits to create new, positive ones. Instead of the second cup of coffee, drink a tall glass of water. Instead of watching another episode of your favourite series, take a walk – even a short one.

We are, by nature, creatures of habit; we prefer to follow the same patterns every day. We tend to wake up at the same time each day, brush our teeth, have morning coffee, and then start our day. Change is hard, and forming healthy habits is even harder, but here are some ways you can start to change your habits and begin to have healthy codes and transform your body.

- For many of us, our morning routine is our strongest routine, so that's a great place to begin to develop a new habit.
- Start small. It has taken me many years of daily practice to incorporate the five codes into my life. Some are easier than others.
- Think about your end-of-the-day habits, as well. Do you tend to flop on the couch after work and turn the TV on? How about making a small change by doing a yoga pose instead, or a breathing exercise, or just close your eyes and think about the day.

Let's face it, habits take a long time to create, but they form faster when we do them more regularly, so start with something reasonable that you find easy to do. You are more likely to stick with an exercise habit if you do some small exercise — jumping jacks, a yoga pose, a brisk walk — every day, rather than trying to get to the gym three days a week.

Once daily exercise becomes a habit, you can explore new, more intense forms of exercise – and then, you are on your way.

Feeling rewarded is an important part of forming a habit. Some rewards are immediate – when you have a good sleep, you wake up refreshed. But some rewards such as weight loss or the body changes from exercise take longer to show. That's why it helps to build in some immediate rewards to help you form the habit. Listening to audiobooks while running, for example, or watching a favourite cooking show on the treadmill can help reinforce an exercise habit. Or plan an exercise date, so the reward is time with a friend.

Remember, change takes time. Some say it takes a minimum of 28 days, and some say it takes 66 days to form a new habit. By focussing on your new habit daily and being consistent, you will definitely see results in coding your body transformation.

The world we live in has made us want instant gratification. We want everything now. We want our online purchases to be delivered today. We want to feel the benefits of weight loss and fitness now. It can't take weeks and months. We don't want to lose grams or 1kg at a time; we want 2-3 kgs to miraculously drop off. We want toned muscles, and we want them now.

Cracking the Body Transformation Code is not about instant gratification and quick results. It is about adopting a focussed lifestyle that consistently keeps you in a state of living well and being fit.

The most challenging aspect of the programme is getting all five codes working together. Of course, it is about breaking habits that keep you locked and releasing you to a new way to see yourself.

I believe that there are no short cuts, but with a positive mindset and introducing the codes in this book into your life, you will be following proven ways to a new you!

To your success!